LAZY
witchcraft
FOR
CRAZY,
sh*tty
DAYS

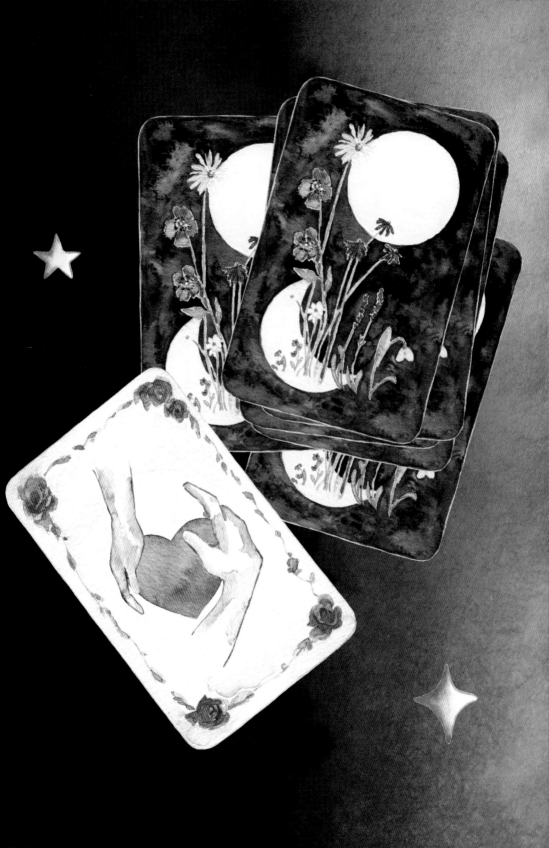

LAZY
witchcraft
FOR
CRAZY,
sh✪tty
DAYS

EASY SPELLS AND RITUALS
FOR WHEN YOU'RE
STRESSED OUT, WIPED OUT, OR JUST
HAVE NO MORE SPOONS TO GIVE

ANDREA SAMAYOA
Creator of Moon Street Kits

FAIR WINDS

Quarto.com
© 2024 Quarto Publishing Group USA Inc.
Text © 2024 Andrea Samayoa
Illustrations © 2024 Kim Crago-Moon

First Published in 2024 by Fair Winds Press, an imprint of The Quarto Group,
100 Cummings Center, Suite 265-D, Beverly, MA 01915, USA.
T (978) 282-9590 F (978) 283-2742

Fair Winds Press titles are also available at discount for retail, wholesale, promotional, and bulk
purchase. For details, contact the Special Sales Manager by email at specialsales@quarto.com or by
mail at The Quarto Group, Attn: Special Sales Manager, 100 Cummings Center, Suite 265-D, Beverly,
MA 01915, USA.

28 27 26 25 24   2 3 4 5

ISBN: 978-0-7603-9264-5

Digital edition published in 2024
eISBN: 978-0-7603-9265-2

Library of Congress Cataloging-in-Publication Data available

Design: Samantha J. Bednarek, samanthabednarek.com
Page Layout: Samantha J. Bednarek, samanthabednarek.com
Illustration: Kim Crago-Moon

Printed in USA

The information in this book is for educational purposes only. It is not intended to replace
the advice of a physician or medical practitioner. Please see your health-care provider before
beginning any new health program.

dedication

I'd like to dedicate this book to
everyone who prayed for my downfall.

No, just kidding, that would be wild.
I'm actually dedicating this to my little
brother, Alex, for being the best support
system I've had throughout this journey.
I quite literally would not have been able
to write this book without him.

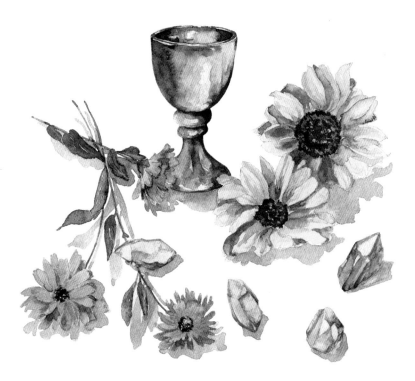

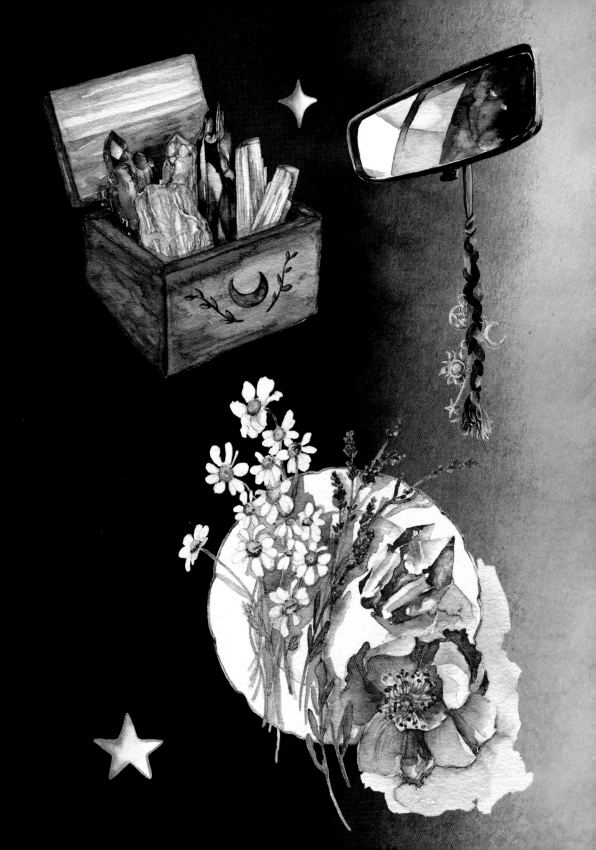

contents

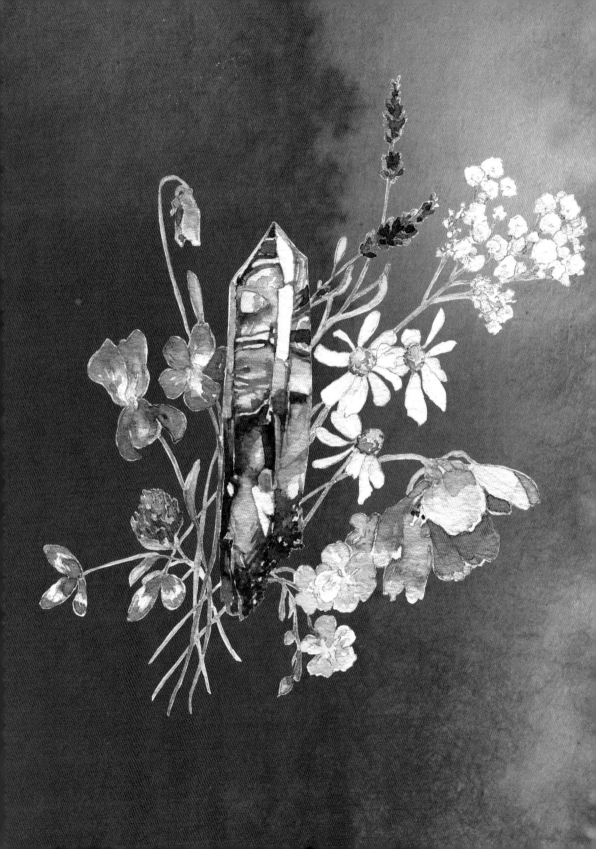

introduction

Welcome to the easiest book of witchcraft that you'll ever find. *Lazy Witchcraft for Crazy, Sh*tty Days* was created for those of us who want to be witchy so bad but can't seem to find the time, energy, or will to live (at least some days). It's for those of us who see all the fascinating, complicated spells and rituals online and think, "That's cute… but it seems like a lot of work." Whether you suffer from an illness that leaves you fatigued or are just so fucking tired from trying to function like a "normal" human is supposed to in our society, this book is here to help. DON'T TAKE IT TOO SERIOUSLY. Are there times we need to be serious? Sure. But this book is not about summoning demons from the underworld to burn down capitalism; it's to help you survive this thing we call life.

Now you're probably wondering, "Why the fuck should I listen to this random ass lady?" So let me give you some background. Hi, I'm Andrea. I started doing spells when I was very young, eventually turning my interest into not just a full-blown spiritual practice but a career, as well. As a practicing witch and owner of the online metaphysical shop Moon Street Kits, I was used to doing magic every single day. Spells, rituals, crafts, literally anything you can think of— until my health intervened.

Out of nowhere, I started feeling tired, unmotivated, and basically overpowered by executive dysfunction. I was eventually diagnosed with anemia, but the medication took a very long time to start working (this is on top of my already-existing anxiety and mental health issues). The one thing that bothered me the most throughout this saga was my inability to practice my witchcraft. I started researching and searching for simpler spells that could meet my low-energy needs and, girl, why the fuck was it still so complicated? Then it hit me. It doesn't need to be. Witchcraft is about intention more than anything, so why does a spell need to have a million ingredients to work? I looked at my *Book of Shadows*, packed with spells I'd developed through years of research and practice, and thought, "I can make this easier." And I did.

Switching to a low-effort, low-energy approach completely changed and revitalized my practice and eventually led to this book. "Lazy witchcraft" means super easy, super low-effort, super low-energy spells and rituals. And "for crazy, shitty days" means for days when you are struggling, whether that be with stress, chronic illness, executive dysfunction, depression, anxiety, or other physical, mental, or emotional health challenges. Because, these days, who isn't?

HOW TO USE THIS BOOK

Each chapter of this book (aside from Chapter One—more on that in a sec) covers a different intention—the reason you're doing the spell in the first place. It could be focus, healing, protection, learning to love your shadow shelf, whatever. If I were you, I'd start in chronological order for the first three chapters. Chapter 1 will give you basics you'll use throughout the book. Chapter 2 will give you a baseline on manifestation since, technically, all spells use manifestation. Chapter 3 is all about protection, which is the most important part of the craft. The last three chapters can be done in any order, depending on what you need on any given day. Struggling with self-worth? Chapter 4 has your back. Got a deadline and can't focus? Hit up Chapter 5. Need some cold, hard cash (don't we all?) see Chapter 6.

At the beginning of each chapter, you'll find a list of correspondences, ingredients, and substitutions. Correspondences are a list of herbs, crystals, colors, etc., that match a certain intention. For example, if your intention is self-love, then some of its correspondences would be pink, rose quartz, and rose petals. Your correspondence tables can also be used to create your own spells once you're comfortable enough and get into the flow of low-energy witchcraft.

Throughout the book, you'll see that all the spells have a "spoon" rating. Spoons are simply a measurement of the amount of energy you have to give in the current moment. I've based this system on a ten-spoon scale. Think of a ten like a full-scale two-day ritual with costumes, feasts, and other wild shit, while a one might be lighting a candle and making a wish. In this book, we're never going over a five, because that's all that most of us can give after we've given so much to work, school, family, and friends.

Before we get started, I'd like to take a moment to throw in some disclaimers. This book was created by me, shaped by my belief system, and based on how I view witchcraft. Each practitioner has his or her own way of doing things since witchcraft is a practice, not a religion. I am not Wiccan, Christian, Jewish, Muslim, or anything else. I have no religion. Incorporating your personal belief system into your craft is a wonderful way to brand your spellwork, which will help make your rituals stronger. I'll be referencing the universe quite a bit throughout the book. The universe is who I pray to, manifest to, and give offerings to. Feel free to switch the term out for whomever you'd like.

Witchcraft doesn't have to be scary or complicated or feel like work. My goal in this book is to make witchcraft as accessible as I possibly can. The spells I give you will be easy and straight to the point, babe. Don't let that little voice in the back of your head stop you from practicing. Whether you're a tenured, seasoned witch or you're just starting out, we all sometimes get this thing called imposter syndrome. Imposter syndrome is when you know exactly what you're doing, but your brain is like, "Nope, you suck. You have no idea what's happening. Please just stop." Yes, it even happens to me. Tell that voice to fuck off.

Ready to do some spells? Let's get started.

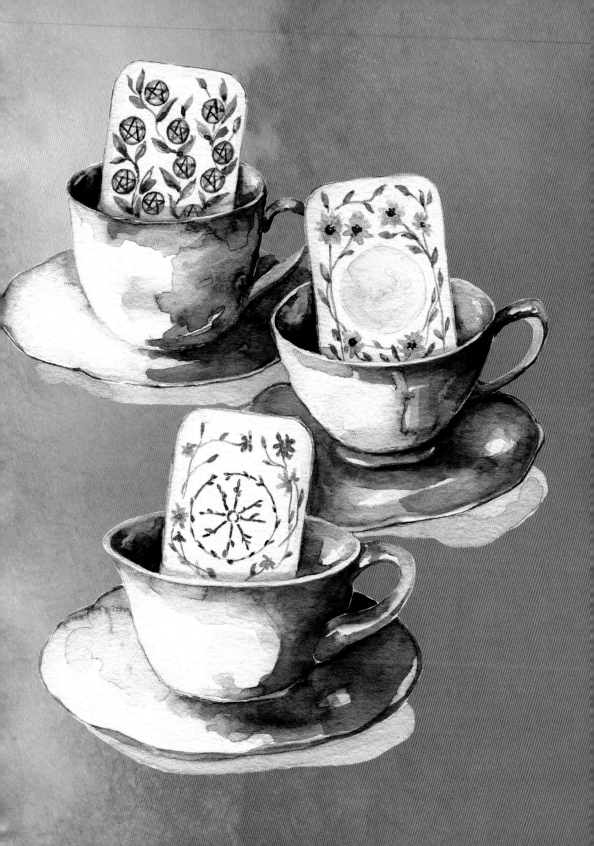

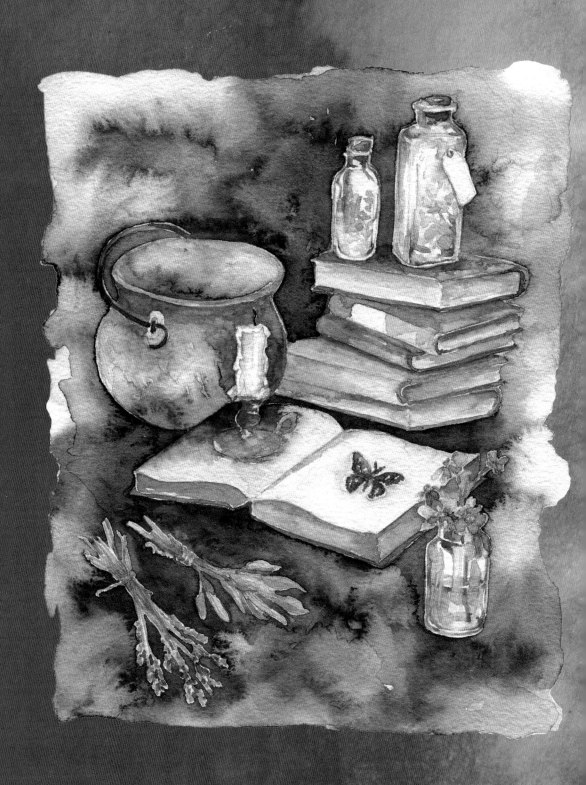

1

what TF
DO I NEED?
+
how TF
DO I DO THIS?

In this first chapter, we'll be covering the tools, practices, and techniques that form the basis of the spells in this book. Some of these you'll probably recognize, but I've added my own "lazy" twist to a lot of it to make it more accessible (while keeping the same energy and intention). In some cases, this is literally just permission to buy the cheaper, easier-to-find version of the item. Witchcraft does not need to cost a lot of money and thrift stores are your friend, babes. Now let's see what the fuck you'll need to do this shit.

what TF
DO I NEED?

Every witch will tell you that you need something different for your spellwork. While I think candles are more important than cauldrons, another witch might say the opposite. The most crucial thing is to remember that the tools are just mundane objects without you. You are divinely connected to the universe; the magic comes from you.

YOUR BASIC LAZY WITCH TOOLKIT

Below is a list of every type of tool you'll use in this book and some alternatives for those of us who don't have easy access to those tools or are still a newbie in the witchy closet (don't worry babe, you got this). Just remember, a tool that costs $100 works just as well as one that you got from the thrift store. Regardless of where you get them, you'll need to cleanse them. I'll show you a few ways to do that further into this chapter.

LIGHTERS

If you want to be super fancy, you can match your lighter color to your intention and candle color, but I didn't write this whole ass book for y'all to be fancy. I wrote it so we could be lazy but still effective. Get yourself to a gas station and grab one of those. If it produces fire, it works.

CHARCOAL

This is not the charcoal you use to light a grill. You're looking for charcoal disks. These are usually easier to buy online since the only shops I've seen carrying charcoal disks are smoke shops, and I'm just going to assume not all of us are comfortable going into certain places. Charcoal disks can stay ignited for four to six hours, but you won't ever need it to be lit that long for this book. Instead, break the charcoal disk into four pieces. This will make it burn for thirty minutes to one hour, which is the perfect amount of time.

TONGS AND TWEEZERS

These are mostly meant to handle your charcoal. When you light charcoal, you have to hold it up to the flame for thirty seconds to two minutes, depending on the quality of the charcoal. Holding it with tongs or tweezers makes life so much easier and creates less stress, as the possibility of burning yourself goes down exponentially.

FIREPROOF VESSELS

If you're burning something in a bowl or on a plate, IT NEEDS TO BE FIREPROOF OR FIRE-RESISTENT. Please, for the love of everything holy and unholy, follow this rule. You can find fireproof incense burners online. The little ramekins that you can bake with? Those are also fireproof. Cast-iron cauldrons are fireproof, as well. A few spells in this book will require you to stick candles to plates; those should also be, you guessed it, fireproof. Remember, fireproof doesn't mean the vessel won't get hot—it most certainly will—so when you're burning anything, make sure the surface isn't made out of plastic. And, of course, never, ever, EVER leave anything burning unattended.

SAND

Always keep sand on your workspace. When we dress candles (more on that later) or light herbs, it produces a fire that can give you high flames. I don't know about y'all, but that shit gives me anxiety. Pouring water on it is fine unless the spell contains oils; but pouring water on fire basically boils the water, which has the potential of splashing you. It's not a good time. But sand? Sand is reliable at dousing any amount of fire. Use sand.

BOWLS

Mixing bowls and ritual bowls don't have to be made out of a certain material. In the witchcraft community. People sometimes frown upon the use of plastic, but they don't take into consideration the simple fact that a lot of people just can't afford nice things. That being said, glass is preferred but not mandatory. If you're ballin' on a budget, go to a thrift store. You can get bowls for $1 that work just as well as the $20 ones you can find at HomeGoods.

CANDLES

There are quite a few types of candles: chime, tealight, pillar, jar, taper, etc. You know what people usually don't tell you to use? Birthday candles. Birthday candles are cheap as fuck and give the same outcome that a $40 candle from the mall gives. Even thrifted candles work just fine. As my own rule, any candle can be switched out for a white candle unless it's a protection spell. Those candles should always be black (in my opinion). So if you only have those two colors, you're good to go.

When dressing your candles, PLEASE BE CAREFUL. Herbs and oils do catch fire, and your candle will absolutely catch fire if the herbs are too big or you add too much oil. If you're not comfy using fire, you can always use battery-powered candles. Paint some Mod Podge on the outside, and drop your herbs on. Let it dry, and there you have it: a fake spell candle that works just as well.

CANDLE HOLDERS

Again, do you need them? Not at all. You can melt the bottom of a chime candle and stick it to a fireproof plate and call it a day. But if you want them, you can get any kind from anywhere. Go nuts, but again... FIREPROOF.

BOTTLES AND JARS

Thrift that shit. Reuse old pasta jars. Keep your old perfume bottles. Empty spice jars? Fucking elite, bitch. You can even reuse spell jars you've already made once the original spell has been completed. I'll show you how to do that later, as well. If you want to be fancy, I usually use 20-milliliter bottles with corks for my spell jars. They're the perfect size. For containers, I use jars and bottles that are meant to store spices and things for the kitchen.

RITUAL SPOONS AND KNIVES

You can get ritual spoons and knives from witchcraft and metaphysical shops, or just go to your kitchen. Does the spoon mix? Great, then it's a witchcraft spoon. Does the knife cut? Great, it's a witchcraft knife now. The only thing I will say is that you shouldn't interchange them. Once you've used something for witchy activities, keep those specifically for that purpose. That way you don't have to worry about cross-contamination. You don't want to add anything to your spells that's not supposed to be there, and you don't want to eat anything from your spells that isn't meant to be ingested.

CARVING TOOLS

We use these tools to carve sigils, symbols, or words into candles. Old pens, vinyl weeders, cuticle pushers—anything that can carve basically. It doesn't have to be super sharp, but you do need something with a point.

PAINT BRUSHES

I know damn well none of you want to be smelling a strong-ass essential oil all fucking day. When you dress candles, using a paint brush to paint it on does two things. One, it allows you to evenly spread it and control the placement and amount that you're putting on your candle. Two, it keeps your hands nice and clean, so you don't get a migraine from smelling some potent-ass shit all day. Gloves are also an option; I just hate how they feel. Probably my low-key neurodivergent brain. If you can relate, grab a paintbrush.

SPELL PAPER

Printer paper, notebook paper, and parchment paper all work for this purpose. I prefer to use handmade paper since I'm usually burning it and some factory-processed papers have chemicals that aren't good to inhale. Well, no smoke is great to inhale, but let's try to keep the exposure to a minimum, right? Handmade paper has a shorter biodegradability time span. Some other planet-friendly options include hemp paper, reclaimed straw, recycled cotton, bamboo, sugarcane, seed paper, and recycled paper.

STRING AND ROPE

Head on over to a craft store and grab the cheapest kind. My favorite to use is twine. I don't know why, but it gives a rustic witchy feel to my spells while also saving me money because twine can be found pretty much everywhere. If you're feeling crafty, (even though we're only using four or five different colors throughout the whole book, generally speaking) you can dye the twine instead of buying fifty different colors of string.

SACHETS AND STRAINERS

Sachets are usually made of a muslin material, making them perfect for spell or charm bags but also tea strainers. Yup, a two-for-one. Muslin is a thin material so putting your tea blends in them and directly brewing them in boiling water works just as well as, if not better than, a strainer. Strainers tend to be metal and have tiny holes in them, which allows powdered herbs like chamomile to seep through. You don't want to be choking mid-spell because a piece of lavender got stuck at the back of your throat. If you want to go extra DIY on your charm bags, you can grab some fabric squares from your local craft store and either sew or simply tie the squares together once your ingredients are inside.

RUBBING ALCOHOL AND WITCH HAZEL

Rubbing alcohol is used throughout this book to stop water spells from molding. You can switch this out for vodka or witch hazel. The only issue I have with substituting in witch hazel is the smell that it gives off. I very much dislike the smell of witch hazel. Rubbing alcohol also has a longer shelf life.

PENS AND MARKERS

I suggest having one pen, one permanent marker, and one paint marker. The pen is for writing on spell paper. Permanent markers work fantastically on bay leaves, and the paint marker works on glass. The writing tools don't need to be specifically used for witchcraft, meaning you can use the same pen that you used to write that love letter to your ex (that you should definitely not fucking send, they're an ex for a reason, babe).

COLORS AND SHIT

Here's a list of colors and their correspondences. Working with the right colors in witchcraft helps enhance our spells and rituals by adding power to our correspondences and amplifying our intentions. Remember, most colors can be substituted with white, the universal absence of color. Of course, there are more correspondences for each color, but if I try to fit them all in here, it'll turn into a novel. Here are the basics.

Colors	Zodiac	Tarot	Intentions
Red	Aries	The Devil	Lust, reversal, passion, strength, fertility
Orange	Virgo	The Hermit	Abundance, creativity, energy, confidence
Yellow	Gemini	The Star	Clarity, communication, inspiration
Green	Pisces	The Empress	Growth, prosperity, money, nature
Blue	Aquarius	The Fool	Intuition, emotions, dreams, purification
Purple	Sagittarius	The Wheel of Fortune	Divination, protection, psychic ability
Pink	Libra	The Lovers	Love, self-love, harmony, warmth
Brown	Taurus	The Hermit	Grounding, balance, success, guidance
White	Capricorn	The High Priestess	Purification, healing, light, all purpose
Black	Scorpio	The World	Banishing, warding, spirituality, protection
Silver	Cancer	The Moon	Beginnings, intuition, lunar magic
Gold	Leo	The Sun	Abundance, creativity, healing, wealth

MOON WATER AND SUN WATER

Moon and sun water are used in various spells throughout the book so we're going to learn how to make them right now. You may think "moon water" and "sun water" sound fancy and complicated, but, actually, they couldn't be easier to make.

For both, you'll need water and a container. The water can be any type; however, if you're going to use it to brew tea or in facial mists, I suggest using bottled or filtered water. Your container can be made of any material. Most witches are obsessed with glass, which is fine but may not be accessible for everyone, so plastic works just fine.

To make moon water, pour water into your container of choice, and leave it outside under direct moonlight from sunset to sunrise.

To make sun water, pour water into your container of choice, and leave it outside from sunrise to sunset.

If you have a hard time remembering things like I do, set an alarm on your phone to tell you when to bring the waters outside and inside. And that's literally it—you're just charging the water outside by the light of the sun or moon.

Each moon phase and solar event has its own set of correspondences (see the chart below). You can choose what phase or event you'd like to make your water with based on its intentions. If you want to get extra technical, you can categorize your sun water by looking at the zodiac sign it is currently in, but we're not about to do all of that for this book.

MOON PHASES AND SOLAR EVENTS

Full Moon	Intuition, psychic abilities, abundance, protection, releasing, grounding
New Moon	Personal growth, manifestation, abundance, fertility, new relationships, grounding, stability
Solar	Energy, strength, healing, happiness, fertility, creativity, inspiration, clarity
Solar and Lunar Eclipses	Banishing, cursing, grounding, protection, transmutation of energy, rejuvenation
Waning Moon	Banishing, rest, renewal, divination, dreams, intuition, healing, communication
Waxing Moon	Success, attraction, communication, balance, organization, intuition, healing

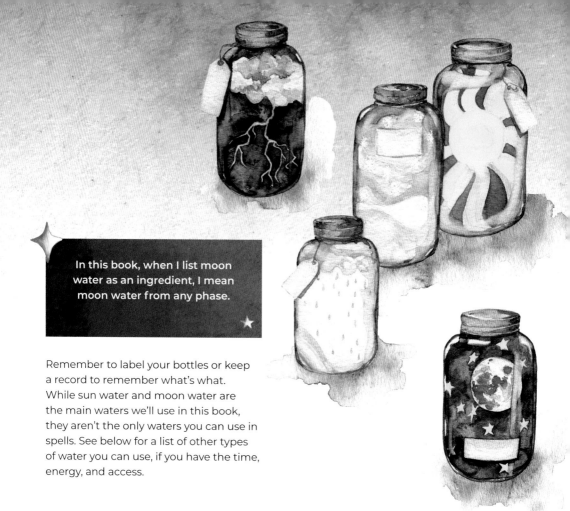

In this book, when I list moon water as an ingredient, I mean moon water from any phase.

Remember to label your bottles or keep a record to remember what's what. While sun water and moon water are the main waters we'll use in this book, they aren't the only waters you can use in spells. See below for a list of other types of water you can use, if you have the time, energy, and access.

OTHER WATERS

Lake	Peace, joy, contentment, relaxation, self-reflection
Rain	Growth, rebirth, cleansing, scrying
River	Moving on, focus, warding, breaking through, power, charging
Sea	Cleansing, protection, balance, healing, manifestation
Snow	Transformation, balance, peace, endings
Storm	Vitality, self-esteem, courage, strength, protection
Well	Healing, wishes, psychic power, manifestation

how TF
DO I DO THIS?

Now that we've got our materials sourced and ready to go, let's talk through some basic rules, techniques, and practices for doing witchcraft. These can be done (and in some cases, *should* be done—cough cough—SET YOUR INTENTIONS) before, after, or in combination with the rest of the spells in this book. Or on their own. It's up to you how you use these practices, but you should work them into your craft somewhere because they make everything work better. Trust me, I'm a lazy witch.

SETTING INTENTIONS

If you've watched any of my content on the Moon Street Kits TikTok page, you know damn well how much of an emphasis I put on setting intentions. It's for a very good reason. You could use all the herbs, crystals, and magical tools in the world, but without intention, you're just making pretty jars and incense that smells good. Intention is the purpose of your spell. Think of it like the universe asking you, "Why the fuck are you doing this shit?" Each herb and crystal should know its purpose and what it's there for. Imagine, for example, you're in a crowded airport, but no one knows when their flight is or what gate they're going to and everything is on fire. That's how your ingredients feel when you stick them in a jar without a purpose.

Setting intentions can be done a few different ways, the most common being a chant, affirmation, or prayer, and sometimes even visualizations. The easiest way is to quite literally tell everything why they're there and what they're doing. For example, let's say you're doing a spell and the ingredients are angelica, rosemary, and hyssop. Do you know the purpose of the spell just from me saying that? Obviously not, because I just made that shit up. YOU NEED TO SET INTENTIONS. Each ingredient has multiple correspondences so pretend they're just as confused as you are.

As I mentioned in the Introduction, correspondences are the intentions that a specific ingredient has. Most ingredients have up to thirty different intentions, which is another reason why we need to be specific when sending our desired intention out into the universe.

Visualization is another form of setting intentions. It's harder than chanting, affirmations, and prayer, but it is SLIGHTLY more effective in the sense that you can visualize exactly what you want and how you see the outcome, which leaves less room for error. Visualizing is best done throughout the entire spell. We don't use visualization much in this book, because I wanted to make everything as easy as possible. But just know you can use it in your witchcraft, if you want to.

As an example, let's imagine we're doing a quick healing spell. You have chamomile, lavender, rose petals, and amethyst that are going into a spell jar. You'd say:

"Chamomile, heal my mind and clear my negative thoughts.
Rose, help me love myself unconditionally, even when it's hard.
Lavender, bring me peace and serenity while keeping me balanced.
Amethyst, transmute all negative energy into positive energy, instead of just getting rid of it."

Setting intentions stops your spells from having unwanted effects or unintended consequences and gives the universe a clear message of what you want. So, if it's all about intentions, why do we need herbs and crystals? Well, technically, you don't. But without them, your intention has to be stronger than it ever has before. Herbs and crystals boost your intentions.

Setting intentions might seem like a lot of work in the beginning, but once you practice, you'll find yourself doing it automatically.

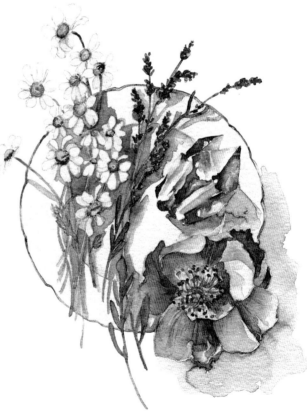

RAISING YOUR VIBRATIONS

Before we get into vibrations, I want to make something super clear. So clear, in fact, I'm going to emphasize it in caps: WITCHCRAFT IS NEVER A RELACEMENT FOR MEDICATION.

I mention this now because some of the symptoms you may experience when you're at a low vibrational frequency could actually be signs of a physical and mundane illness. Please always consult with a medical professional before assuming you can fix something with witchcraft.

Your vibration is your own personal frequency that is controlled by your emotions, thoughts, and feelings. It's similar to your aura, but vibrations are more in the moment. To me, auras are an overall representation of you as a human. They're more fixed, while your vibrations change frequently, almost with every thought you have.

When we raise our vibrations, we're raising the frequency with which we go about our daily lives. How do we know if our vibrations are low? You'll feel it. Symptoms include:

- Tiredness
- Low motivation
- Aches
- Clouded thoughts
- Negative self-talk
- Depression
- Anxiety
- Fatigue
- Migraines
- An overall sense of despair

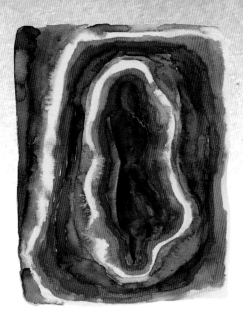

By contrast, when your vibrations are high, you feel energetic, at peace, and generally happier to be alive. Guess which one is best for doing witchcraft?

When your vibration is low, you become (for lack of a better term) a breeding ground for bad energy. When you have high vibrations, you are more likely to attract positive energy, which is what we want when we're doing spells. Here are a few easy suggestions for how to raise those vibrations and invite positive things to come into your life.

BREATHE, BITCH
This will make you feel more energized, calmer, and more connected the universe and its energy.

HUG A PERSON

Hugging helps stimulate the release of oxytocin in the body. Oxytocin relaxes the nervous system, reduces stress, strengthens the immune system, improves heart health, and improves overall well-being.

PRACTICE GRATITUDE

Focus on the things in your life that you are grateful for. This can help you channel your energy into a more positive state.

DO ACTIVITIES THAT MAKE YOU HAPPY

Activities that you enjoy and bring you peace can help raise your vibration by increasing positive emotions.

GO OUTSIDE

The earth keeps us grounded and in the moment, which brings clarity and helps lower anxiety. Walking outside barefoot and (literally) hugging trees—grounding—does wonders for the soul. We'll go deeper into grounding in the next section of this chapter.

MEDITATE

I know, I know, I know. Sitting and doing nothing for extended periods of time is so annoying and often impossible for my neurodivergent humans out there. You can use a guided meditation audio from any online source, if that helps. If not, did you know dancing is meditation? Washing dishes? Zen coloring books? Laying down and listening to music? All of these are forms of mediation because they're easy and repetitive and give our mind something to focus on so our subconscious can have a turn in the limelight. Find an activity you do regularly and see if that works for you instead. Personally, I paint.

ACTS OF KINDNESS

Helping others makes us feel good inside. I know it, you know it, and the old lady crossing the street alone during rush hour will appreciate it either way.

AFFIRMATIONS

Affirmations are phrases made to motivate you and set intentions. You can find tons of affirmations online for anything in your life. Repeating affirmations helps build that thought up in our heads, basically low-key gaslighting yourself until it becomes a reality. One of my favorite techniques for this is to grab a dry erase marker and write affirmations on mirrors, windows, the refrigerator, wherever (as long as it's erasable). This lets you switch the affirmations out quickly and easily.

CRYSTALS

Laying down and placing crystals on your body helps raise your vibrations by infusing your energy with the energy from said crystal. You can place your favorites all over your body or create a personal system that works for you. I use rose quartz on my heart to build self-love. Labradorite on my forehead to open the third eye. Obsidian on my tummy because your girl is allergic to dairy and we need to protect it from that, trust me. Use whatever crystals you have and whatever feels right to you.

CLEANSING

Cleansing and purifying are basically the same thing in my eyes. When you cleanse yourself, you're getting rid of all the nasty ass shit that's gotten stuck to you spiritually. Think of it like a spiritual shower: you cleanse yourself so your energies aren't blocked and grimy when you're doing your spells. You also need to cleanse your tools. This removes all residual energies from spells you've performed in the past, so you don't contaminate your current spell.

Whatever you're cleansing and however you're choosing to cleanse (see below), it's important to hold your intention throughout your cleansing ritual. Stay as focused as you can. I also recommend following up your cleansing activities by filling the space or infusing the tool (see below) or yourself with positive energy to avoid negative energies from coming back in.

Here are some ways to cleanse:

CRYSTALS

Selenite and clear quartz are natural healers and chargers. You can cleanse yourself with these crystals by simply holding them and letting all that muddy energy leave you and seep into the crystal instead. You can cleanse your tools with crystals by placing them on top of or underneath the crystals.

SOUND

There are different specific sound frequencies that we know are cleansing, but your favorite song? That's perfect as a personal cleanser. Choose a song that brings happiness or good core memories. Blast it, and feel immediately better.

SMOKE

Smoke is pretty much everyone's go-to method for cleansing. You can light incense and cleanse a whole space with it or just a small jar or other tool. If you're a smoker of the green stuff, that smoke can also be used to cleanse. If you're using incense, stick to scents that have cleansing or purification correspondences. Some of my favorites include Sandalwood, Rosemary, and Cedar.

SALT

Salt soaks up negative energy. Sprinkle it on your tools or in your space and let it do its work. Discard in the trash when done. NEVER pour salt directly on the earth; it dehydrates it and nothing will ever grow on that spot again.

WATER

Water is an obvious cleanser, not only in the mundane world, but also in the metaphysical world. You can visualize water cleansing yourself as you drink it or as you shower.

SUNLIGHT AND MOONLIGHT

We discussed the correspondences for these on page 19, but they can also be used as powerful cleansers. Sit outside under either to cleanse yourself or leave your tools out and cleanse those instead.

How often you cleanse is absolutely up to you, but I personally do it every time I physically clean my house; this just makes it easier for my brain to remember.

A GENERAL HOME CLEANSING RITUAL

YOUR HOME SHOULD be spiritually cleansed at least once a month. That's not to say you can't cleanse more often than that. If you feel any sort of negativity or "heavy" energy in your space, you can use this ritual to clear it out.

In this ritual, we'll use floor salts to absorb all the negative energy in a room. I haven't listed specific amounts (tablespoons, cups, etc.) for any of the herbs, because I want you to be able to make as much or as little of the salt mix as you need. However, do pay attention to the ratios, as that can make a difference.

4 parts sea salt

1 part lavender

1 part chamomile

1 part rosemary

1 part cinnamon

1 part patchouli

20 to 30 drops of lavender or lemon essential oil (optional)

Mixing bowl

Before cleansing your space spiritually, start with the mundane. Pick up any clutter, wipe off counters, organize clutter. But don't sweep—we'll do that later.

To make your floor salts, combine all of your ingredients into a mixing bowl. As you add them, tell them why they're here.

Salt, you'll be absorbing and trapping the negative energy in my space.
Lavender and chamomile, you'll be adding peace and calming energy to replace it.
Rosemary, you'll be cleansing the negative energy.
Cinnamon, you'll be creating a barrier once all the negative energy is gone.
Patchouli, you'll be transforming the negative energy into positive energy.

Mix the ingredients with your hands and (stay with me, bitch) toss it all over your floors. You don't need to use a ton and cover every inch of your floor; a light sprinkle will do the trick.

Let the salt sit on your floor for ten to fifteen minutes before sweeping. Make sure you're sweeping from the back of the house and pushing the pile out of the front door. If you use a vacuum, vacuum in the same direction, but make sure you dump the contents of your vacuum outside of your home when you've finished.

Now you have a clean slate to work with, which ensures your spell is free from outside metaphysical contaminants.

GROUNDING AND CENTERING

Grounding, also known as centering, is a practice that has been around for thousands of years. The earth has a healing vibration all on its own, and when we ground, we absorb that energy, which, in turn, helps us feel peace, clarity, and a sense of overall well-being. When you're "ungrounded," your energy flow is basically blocked, which causes your spells to be less powerful or even not work at all.

Grounding connects us back to our original creator and sustainer, the earth. When we do spells and rituals, we use a good amount of energy, since our energy is what powers spells. When we ground before spellwork, we boost that energy, and when we ground after, we renew that energy.

How do we ground? There's a million ways, but I'll just mention my two favorites.

You won't need to ground every time you do a spell (unless you have the energy to), but I do suggest doing it routinely about one to two times a month.

NATURE WALKING

I referenced this type of grounding in the vibrations section earlier. It's my favorite because it's so simple. Going outside to a park, the ocean, or even your backyard helps you connect to nature and the earth. You can take it a step further and walk around barefoot, but be careful if you're in a public place, because you never know what's on the ground. Touch the soil or sand. It's really that easy. Gardening is also a great hobby for this reason.

TREE GROUNDING

You probably think I'm about to tell you to go hug a tree, right? Nope. This one is for my people who can't go outside or don't have access to a safe space out in the world. You're literally going to visualize yourself as a tree. Don't laugh. I see you, just hear me out.

First, close your eyes. I'm actually one of those weirdos who cannot visualize with my eyes closed. My daydreams only happen when my eyes are open, so if that's the case for you, ignore me every time I tell you to close your eyes throughout this book; you're totally normal.

Next, visualize yourself outside, standing in a field while barefoot. What do you see? How does it smell? Can you feel a breeze? Is it hot? Cold? By identifying all of these things, you'll be able to visualize more clearly.

Now, pretend there are roots growing from your feet. What color are they? Which direction are they taking? Are they soft or hard? What kind of tree are you?

Imagine the roots digging into the ground and the feel of cool, wet soil. Keep them growing until they're connected to the center of the earth. Finish your tree grounding by thanking the earth.

HOW TO MAKE A SIGIL

What the fuck are sigils? They're symbols made of intentions. Often used in spells and rituals, they can also be used simply to infuse an object or person with the intention the sigil represents. Think of it as your own, personal rune, designed by you, for your own purposes. You can draw, add, or place sigils in any number of places. Some of my favorite places to hide sigils include:

- Doors
- Mirrors
- Notebooks
- On your body
- Shoes
- Clothing
- Under desks
- On tests
- In the air
- Inside your phone case
- In wallets
- Under your doormat
- Bookmarks and books

We'll use these a lot throughout this book, so in this section I'll show you the basic bitch way of creating a sigil. Don't be intimidated by the process. Once you get used to it, the process becomes easier. And if it doesn't, there are sigil generators online that work just as well.

1 Pick an intention. As an example, I'll use PURIFICATION. Next, get rid of all vowels and repeating letters. We're left with PRFCTN. Use the chart below to find the corresponding number that matches each letter you have left over.

For our example, P=6; R=8; F=6; C=3; T=0; N=4. That gives us 686304.

SIGIL LETTER/NUMBER CHART

1	2	3	4	5	6	7	8	9	0
A	B	C	D	E	F	G	H	I	J
K	L	M	N	O	P	Q	R	S	T
U	V	W	X	Y	Z				

Note: Some people don't use the number zero when making this chart, but I do, and this is my book so that's how I'm going to show you.

2 Draw a circle and add the numbers 0-9 inside the circle in a random order. Feel free to copy mine below if you want; the order of the numbers doesn't matter. You can create a new circle for every sigil you make, or do this once and use it for everything. It's up to you and how you want to use your spoons.

What you're doing here is connecting the numbers. Start with your first letter and draw a straight line from it to the next letter. In our example, 6(P) will connect to 8(R).

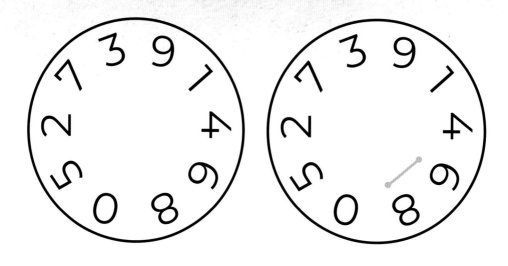

3 Continue connecting the numbers in order until you get to the last number. The last number will connect back to the first. In my example, the 4 connects back to the 6. At this point, your drawing will look something like this:

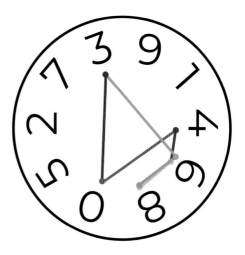

4. The drawing you've made in the circle represents the basic shape of your sigil. Redraw it outside of the circle lower on the page. Mine looks something like this:

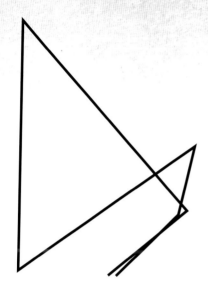

5. This is the fun part. You get to dress it up however you want. Add squiggles, dots, arrows, moons, spirals, circles—anything you want that feels right to you. It doesn't have to be pretty; it just needs to capture your intention. Keep adding and adjusting until you're satisfied, and there you go. You made a motherfucking sigil, y'all.

6. Now, if you're not using your sigil in a specific spell, you need to activate it the first time to get the magic flowing. (I suggest recording your activated sigils in a journal so you can use them more than once.) Copy your sigil onto a paper or bay leaf, and burn it. If fire isn't your thing, bury it. And that's it! Your sigil is activated and ready to use.

Now that we've covered most of the basics, we'll move on to the last, most important basic you'll need for this book. This basic is so fucking important it gets an entire chapter all to itself: manifestation.

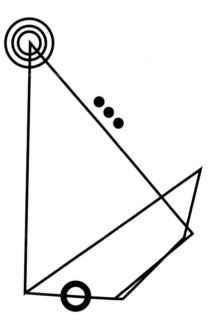

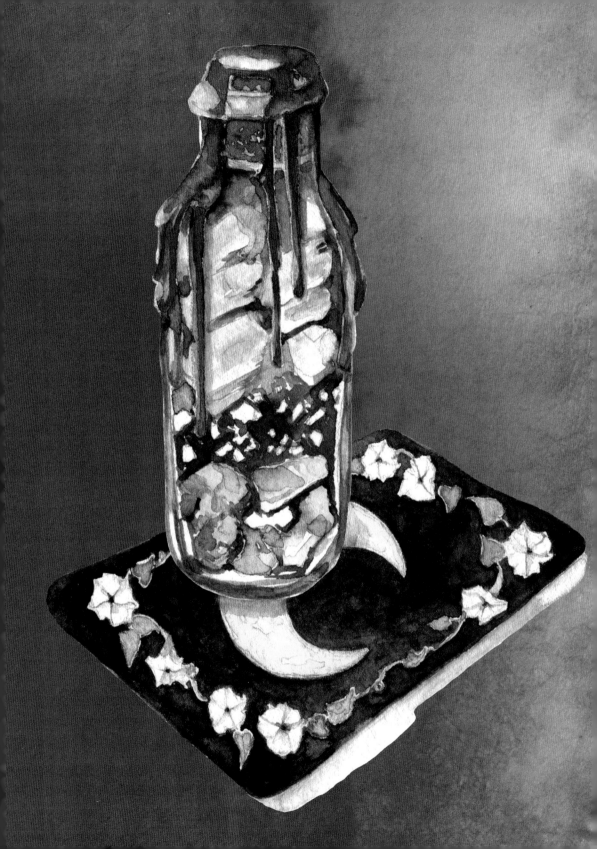

2

THE EASIEST MANIFESTATION
you'll ever do

The basis of all spells is manifestation. Manifestation is the process by which we bring our intentions into fruition, based on the premise that your thoughts create your reality. This idea comes up a lot in the witchcraft world. Positive thoughts equal a positive life, right? But babe, most of us are mentally drained. How are you supposed to "stay positive" and think your dreams into reality when you literally don't want to do anything anymore? How do you manifest when you're having a crazy, shitty day?

The truth is, you don't have to be a positive ray of fucking sunshine 24/7 to manifest or do any spells. That's unrealistic and just wild to say. Instead, we want to try to channel the energy we do have into recognizing the thought patterns that block our manifestations from reaching the universe. We want to be able to say, "Yes, everything is on fire, but, bitch, I got this."

In this chapter, you'll learn the "lazy-unhinged-semi-depressed-anxious-feeling kinda ill" way of manifesting, so you don't get trapped in a cycle of toxic positivity just to try to make your spells work. You can be sad, tired, or angry and still have success when manifesting. The key is using the right tools to amplify your spellwork during those times when you don't feel 100 percent. One of the best tools you can use for this? The moon.

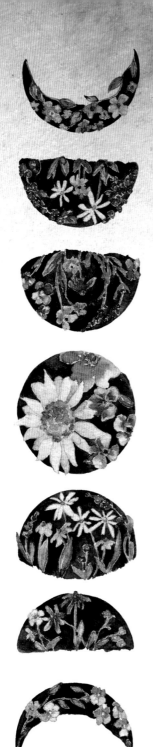

The moon and manifestation are intimately related. If I'm performing a manifestation ritual, you can bet the lunar phase will be a strong point in the spell. The moon is important when manifesting because the phases it cycles through mimic the phases of life, so pairing your intention with the correct phases amplifies the shit out of it. Although the meaning of each moon phase varies, we'll concentrate on the new moon and the full moon in this chapter. The full moon covers abundance, creativity, divination, emotions, energy, fertility, inspiration, magic, protection, psychic ability, and wisdom. The new moon covers beauty, new beginnings, divination, illumination, improvement, optimism, rebirth, relationships, self-work, and stability.

Most of the spells in this chapter are flexible. They don't specify an intention, because they can adapt to any manifestation. I highly recommend combining what you learn in this chapter with spells from other chapters. This will supercharge your intentions for those spells without you having to do much extra work, and that's literally the reason you picked this book up, right? (If you bought it just because you like me then I love you too, babe, but pay attention.)

I'll end this little intro with a relevant quote that I love: *"What you think, you become. What you feel, you attract. What you imagine, you create."* —Buddha

LAZY WITCH TIPS FOR SUCCESSFUL MANIFESTING

When manifesting, it's super important to choose the right words. You want to be as specific as you can (but, remember, be realistic, you're not manifesting marrying Ryan Reynolds—sorry) and you want to keep it in present tense. Instead of using terms like "I want" use "I have" as if its already happened. While manifesting, visualize what your life will look like after the manifestation has already come to fruition. The more detail you can give to the universe, the easier it will be for it to recognize your true goal. Consider the following questions to help you with this:

- What does my life look like after this manifestation?
- Do I look the same? My hair? My skin? My body?
- Do I still have the same people in my life? Is there a new person?
- What does my home look like? Did I move? Did I do home improvements?
- What does my new routine look like?
- Am I in the same job? Same company?
- Do I have the same hobbies? Will I find something new to fill my time?

If you ask yourself these questions and questions like it, your intention will grow exponentially stronger. You know what also helps with manifestation? Fucking confidence. When you believe it will happen, it more than likely will. Try using these affirmations in the morning or before doing a manifestation spell.

- I think highly of myself and am deserving of respect and love.
- I view obstacles as chances for development and achievement.
- I make confident, well-informed decisions because I believe in my intuition.
- I draw good things into my life, and I am worthy of all the good things that come my way.
- I have the ability to get past challenges and use them as stepping stones to achieve my objectives.
- I exude confidence everywhere I go and am at ease in my own skin.
- I recognize my strengths and am proud of my accomplishments.
- I have something special to offer the world in the form of my unique perspective.
- I accept my flaws and understand that they don't make me less valuable.
- I have faith in my skills.

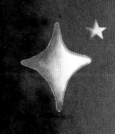

MATERIALS AND CORRESPONDENCES FOR LAZY WITCH
manifestation

The following table shows correspondences for manifestation work and for working with the Full and New Moon.

CORRESPONDENCES FOR MANIFESTATION WORK

	Manifestation (The Intention)	The Full Moon
Moon Phase	Full	Full
Zodiac	Capricorn	Cancer
Day of the Week	Friday	Friday
Colors	Purple, violet, gold, green, orange, pink	Blue, gray, green, orange, silver, white, black
Tarot Card	Hierophant, Magician, The World, The Lovers	The High Priestess, The Moon, The Chariot
Herbs, Plants, and Flowers	Chamomile, lavender, rose, vervain, myrrh, patchouli, sandalwood, cherry bark, basil, jasmine, passionflower, rose, rosemary, yarrow, cinnamon, frankincense, orris root	Sandalwood, jasmine, frankincense, gardenia, rose, orris, ambergris, lotus, violet, myrrh, lemon balm, willow bark, poppy seed, rue, rosemary, passionflower, eucalyptus
Crystals and Gemstones	Amethyst, apatite, blue lace agate, carnelian, citrine, garnet, hematite, lapis lazuli, labradorite, obsidian, tiger's eye, tourmaline, pyrite	Moonstone, clear quartz, smoky quartz, obsidian, hematite, angelite, morganite, selenite

And here is a list of everything
we'll use in this chapter and their substitutions.

The New Moon

New

Libra

Monday

Black, silver, white, pink

The Moon, The Chariot

Vervain, calendula, skullcap, red clover, chamomile, lemon balm, lavender, lemon peel, myrrh, orris root, frankincense, passionflower, rosemary, lotus, gardenia

Clear quartz, peacock ore, citrine, moonstone, lapis lazuli, obsidian

PLANTS, HERBS, AND FLOWERS

Ingredient	Substitution
Bay leaf	Spell paper
Black salt	Sea salt
Cherry bark	Galangal root
Cinnamon	Clove
Eucalyptus	Peppermint
Frankincense	Myrrh
Lemon balm	Lemongrass
Orris root	Rosemary
Passionflower	Yarrow
Pink salt	Sea salt
Rose	Jasmine
Sandalwood	No substitute
Sea salt	Table salt
Vervain	Rue
Willow bark	Cherry bark
Yarrow	Elderflower

When we're doing spells—manifestations, specifically—the best form a crystal can be in is raw. Raw chunks or points. If you only have tumbles, don't freak out and think you need to leave the house and get new ones. Who the fuck wants to do that? Not I, babe, so I wouldn't make you do it either. Tumbles and polished stones work just as well. The raw just allows the energy to flow more effortlessly.

CRYSTALS AND GEMSTONES

Ingredient	Substitution
Amethyst	Garnet
Blue lace agate	Angelite
Clear quartz	No substitute
Labradorite	Amethyst
Moonstone	Labradorite
Obsidian	Tourmaline
Pyrite	Selenite
Rose quartz	Clear quartz
Selenite	Pyrite

CARRIER OILS AND ESSENTIAL OILS

Ingredient	Substitution
Fractionated coconut oil	Olive oil
Gardenia essential oil	Chamomile essential oil
Jasmine essential oil	Jasmine herb, rose essential oil
Olive oil	Coconut oil
Sandalwood essential oil	Sandalwood powder, jasmine essential oil

If you don't have a specific essential oil, you can switch it with the raw herb and vice versa. Never use essential oils directly on the skin, and make sure your pets don't go near them either.

BASIC OILS AND BLENDS FOR
manifestation work

In this chapter, we'll use two different oil blends to boost our manifestation work. These oils appear in multiple spells throughout the chapter, and they are made with the same process. Make them both at the same time, and save your future self some trouble. Of course, you're always more than welcome to use these oils outside of the spells in this chapter. Add them to baths, anoint your pressure points, dress candles, anoint crystals or tools— basically anything you can think of.

MANIFEST THAT SHIT OIL AND LA LUNA OIL

MANIFEST THAT SHIT OIL

THIS MANIFESTATION OIL blend will not only assist in empowering your intention, it also will help you connect to your intuition and link you to a higher power.

2-teaspoon (10-ml) dropper bottle

Cherry bark

Yarrow

Cinnamon

Orris root

Tiny clear quartz points (small enough to fit in the dropper bottle)

Sandalwood essential oil

Fractionated coconut oil

LA LUNA OIL

THIS OIL WILL connect you to the moon and all its powers. It's useful for divination as well as manifestation. The moon is also connected to the water, which is linked to our emotions, making this oil super versatile.

2-teaspoon (10-ml) dropper bottle

Rose

Jasmine

Willow bark

Moonstone chips (small enough to fit in the dropper bottle)

Gardenia essential oil

Olive oil

Cleanse your jars before doing anything else, bitch. (See page 23.) You know damn well you were about to skip that part. I see you.

To make either oil, start by adding your herbs. When you add each herb, repeat the affirmation associated with the oil you're making. The order in which you add them has absolutely no bearing on anything, so do what you fucking want.

For Manifest That Shit Oil, say: *"When I release any resistance and allow the universal energy to flow through me freely, my manifestations come to fruition."* For La Luna Oil, say: *"I am a divine being connected to the infinite wisdom of the moon."*

Once the herbs are in, add your crystals or crystal chips. Repeat the affirmation again.

Last, add 15 to 30 drops of your essential oil in your bottle. The amount depends on how potent you want the smell to be since some humans are more sensitive to scents than others. If you want to be magical about it, use exactly 22 drops.

Fill the rest of your bottle with its corresponding carrier oil. Remember to leave space for the cap because you don't want it to overflow. Cap the bottle and, now, it's time to charge.

For the Manifest That Shit Oil: Leave it on your windowsill or outside for a full twenty-four hours. We want both the sun and the moon to charge it.

For the La Luna Oil: Leave it on your windowsill or outside for one night. You'll want to set it out once the sun goes down and bring it in before the sun comes up. Set an alarm; you'll be fine.

Note: The crystal chips/points in these oils must be tiny enough to fit in the dropper bottle.

When I refer to pressure points, I mean the places where you'll place your oils when you use them on your body. These are your wrists, temples, ankles, bottoms of feet, third eye, and above the belly button, behind your neck, and behind your ears. You never need to use more than a drop unless you're feeling wild.

LUNAR MANIFESTATION INCENSE AND HERB BLEND

WE WILL USE this herb blend, which also functions as an incense, in several spells throughout the chapter. A highly versatile blend, you can use it to enhance spell sachets or charm bags, dress candles, sprinkle around your space, activate sigils (see page 31), or as an offering to your guides or the universe in general.

Rose

Vervain

Sandalwood powder

Eucalyptus

Jasmine essential oil

Mortar and pestle

Container (for storing)

Moonstone or clear quartz (optional)

Combine all of your herbs in your mortar and pestle, and grind them together until you're satisfied with the texture. It does not need to be a fine powder; you just want to get it blended enough that each pinch has a little bit of everything in it. While you're grinding, stay focused on your intention for this blend.

Add in 5 to 10 drops of your essential oil and keep blending. You want the essential oil to touch each component, but you don't want to soak it.

Once your mixture is nice and blended, place both hands over it (one on top of the other) and recite the following: *"Mystic moon and magic herbs, may all intentions that pass through this incense be amplified with your power. Like the water controlled by our lunar goddess, the magic flows through me gently and smoothly. So, mote it be."*

Transfer to your storage container. You can add a piece of moonstone or clear quartz to the container to help keep your herb blend charged.

Note: I'll hardly ever give you exact measurements for your spells in this book, unless it's a tea or something else where the taste/smell matters. Other than that, you'll have to feel it in your soul. There are no wrong answers here; this is your craft.

LAZY WITCH SPELLS FOR
manifestation

NEW MOON CANDLE SPELL

THE NEW MOON brings us the darkest night of the month. Lighting a candle during this moon phase helps bring in a little more illumination into your life.

Carving tool

1 white candle

Sandalwood essential oil

Paintbrush or gloves

Sandalwood powder

The first step in this spell is to make a sigil (see page 29) out of the word LIGHT. Carve it into your candle.

Dab a few drops of sandalwood essential oil on a paint brush. Paint it onto your candle. If you don't have a paint brush, I suggest grabbing some gloves because essential oils are strong and the scent will remain on your hands for quite a while. I don't know about you, but that gives me the worst migraines.

Sprinkle powdered sandalwood all over the candle, making sure to avoid getting it close to the wick.

Light your candle on the new moon, and let it burn all the way down. This spell brings light to your life, which in turn brings joy, happiness, security, and an overall feeling of warmth and love. Use this time to journal and set new intentions for the month.

THE MOON "INTENTION SUPERCHARGER" TAROT SPELL JAR

WITH THIS SPELL, you'll be able to amplify one intention of your choice to help it reach whoever or whatever you pray to.

1 jar with cork

The Moon Tarot Card (see note)

Jasmine

Frankincense

Cinnamon

Vervain

Moonstone chips

Labradorite chips

Pyrite sand

Paper

Pen

1 silver candle (substitute: white)

Before you begin, place your empty jar on top of the tarot card, and let it sit for about two minutes. Use this time to connect with the tarot card and jar. Place your hands around both and close your eyes. Let your energy flow from your hands into your tools.

Add your herbs to the jar followed by the crystal chips. Add them to the jar one at a time, in the following order, telling each one why they're there as you go:

"Jasmine, connect me to the lunar energies.
Frankincense, bless this jar.
Cinnamon, protect my intention from outside forces.
Vervain, amplify my intent to its full potential.
Moonstone, grant me guidance and wisdom.
Labradorite, grant me energy and clarity.
Pyrite, grant me luck and success."

Once all of your ingredients have been added to the jar, it's time to write. Write down your desired outcome on your paper. Keep it to one line for this spell; think of it more like a wish than a manifestation. Roll your paper as small as you can get it, and stick it inside the jar.

Light your candle and seal your jar by dripping wax over the cork. I highly suggest keeping the jar in an area that connects to your manifestation. If you're manifesting business success, keep it in your work space. If you're manifesting love, keep it in the bedroom. If you're manifesting beauty, keep it on your vanity. If you're manifesting happiness, keep it in the kitchen. (The tarot card will stay under the jar the entire time.)

Recharge the spell jar under the full moon once a month until the spell is completed and the manifestations become reality.

Note: If you don't want to sacrifice your moon tarot card for the entirety of this spell, you can print one out and use that instead.

BAY LEAF SIMPLE MANIFESTATION SPELL

THIS IS OUR OG manifestation spell because it can be adapted to any intention or manifestation you have. The key component in the spell is bay leaf, which has been used by the metaphysical world for wishing spells throughout history. This spell is so simple that there's literally no way to mess it up. Make it a mini ritual by adding candles, crystals, or your favorite music.

Charcoal

Charcoal incense burner

Bay leaf (or more—one for each intention)

Lunar Manifestation Incense (see page 41)

Pen

Tweezers

Begin by lighting your charcoal and placing it in your charcoal burner. Take a pinch of your incense and set it on top of the charcoal so it starts to smoke.

Pass your bay leaf through the smoke three times.

Once the leaf has been cleansed by the smoke, draw a sigil symbolizing your intention on the leaf (see page 29 for how to create a sigil). If sigils seem like too much work right now, sum up your manifestation into one word and write that instead. If you have more than one intention, use multiple bay leaves. There should only be one per leaf.

Once your bay leaves have been imbued with your intention, it's time to burn them.

Grab a leaf with your tweezers so you don't burn your fingers and light one end with your lighter. As it burns, think of the details of your manifestation. After the flames hit the halfway point, toss it in your charcoal burner. The charcoal will finish the job for you.

Repeat this process for each bay leaf.

Use the ashes for black salt (see sidebar below) or discard the ashes outside on a windy day.

As black salt is the combination of charcoal or ash with salt, it is not suitable for ingestion. When it comes to protection, black salt is a staple in the witchcraft community. Make your own black salt by adding ashes (from any spell in this chapter) or activated charcoal to a salt of your choice and mixing.

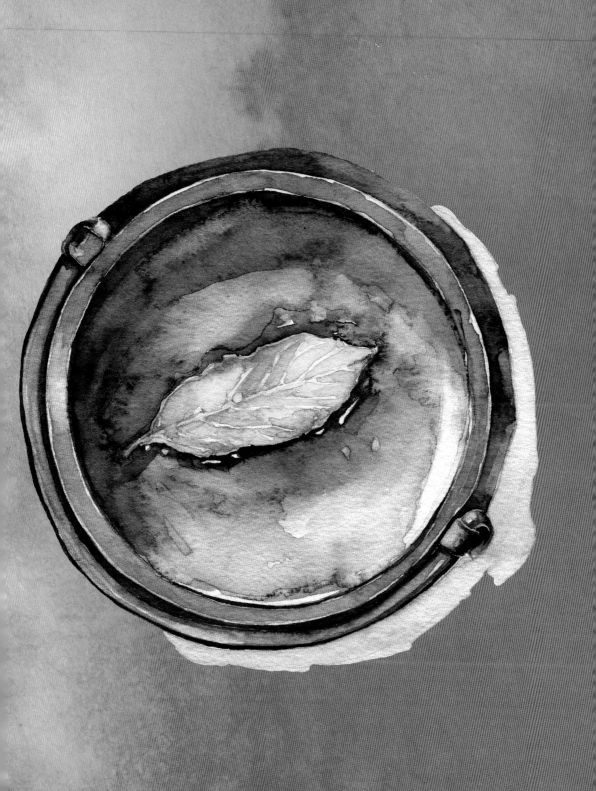

MANIFESTATION CANDLE SPELL

THIS IS ANOTHER very flexible manifestation spell that hinges on the use of one main herb. Which herb? Depends on your intent, babe. You can find herbs and their matching intentions at the beginning of each chapter.

1 purple chime candle

Manifest That Shit Oil (see page 39)

Lunar Manifestation Herb Blend (see page 41)

An intentional herb of your choice

Plate or candleholder

1 moonstone

1 clear quartz

1 amethyst

Paper and pen

Rub your oil on the candle, avoiding the wick (which would be a fire hazard). Then grab your herb blend, add a tiny bit of your intentional herb of choice, and sprinkle a little bit on top of the oil. The oil should make it stick. Place the candle on your work space (use a plate or candleholder), wash your hands, and light the candle. Arrange your crystals in a triangle formation around the base.

Now, it's time to write, bitches. Use your paper and pen to write down your intentions for this spell. To make your life easier, you can answer these questions:

What is your intention?
What do you need to do to get to that intention?
Are there obstacles? How will you get around those?
What does your life look like after the spell has manifested?
What did the manifestation affect in your life?

When you're done, fold the paper toward you once to bring the manifestation in, then fold it twice away from you, to send the manifestation out into the universe.

Burn one of the corners of your paper with the flame of your dressed candle to activate it. Set the singed, folded paper down in front of the candle and wait for the candle to burn all the way down.

Once the candle has burnt out, place your paper under your pillow. (Tap the burned part off really well so you don't have ash all over your sheets.) Before bed, read the manifestation you wrote on the paper out loud three times. When you wake up, read it three more times. Do this for three days.

On the third day, you can either burn the paper completely or you can rip up the paper and discard the ashes in running water.

MANIFESTATION GOALS JOURNAL

WHAT IS MANIFESTATION journaling? Just like every other spell we've done up until this point, it's writing down your hopes, dreams, goals, wishes, and aspirations on a piece of paper—or, in this case, a bunch of pieces of paper, in a book. With this journal, you can work on your manifestations every day, without having to do spellwork every day. Manifestation journaling uses the law of attraction in conjunction with witchcraft to help you manifest whatever it is you want in life.

The spoon rating for this journal starts at two spoons, but the more work you put into it, the more spoons it will take—it's up to you. No two journals will be the same, so whatever you've got to put into it is what it is. I'll help you get started with a bunch of different ideas to set up your journal, ways to decorate it, and thoughts about what to write, but whatever you choose to do is ultimately up to you. Don't let this stress you out at all. It doesn't have to be completed in one day, and it doesn't have to be aesthetically pleasing to anyone else except you. You might think, "Damn, that's a lot of explanation for a lazy witch." And, yeah, you're so right. I'm trying to be as specific as I can, so you don't make anything more complicated than it needs to be.

THE JOURNAL
Choosing your journal should be fairly easy. I suggest going with something that can lay flat so you can journal in bed and still be comfy. You can use any type of notebook; mine is a hardcover I found at TJ Maxx—it's not that serious. Make sure there are over one hundred pages, though, because you'll need to redo the blessing ritual for every new journal you start. And, hello, this is lazy witchcraft.

THE RITUAL
Once you've acquired your journal, it's time to do the ritual (turn the page, babe).

ZERO-SPOON *spell*

Ask an orange a yes-or-no question before you eat it, then count the seeds. If there are an even number of seeds, the answer is no. If there are an odd number of seeds, the answer is yes.

Lunar Manifestation Incense (see page 41)

Manifest That Shit Oil (see page 39)

1 white tealight candle

Journal

Pen or marker

Clear quartz

Find a nice, quiet space. Make sure you have at least ten to fifteen minutes of alone time. (Just tell your significant other and/or kids that you ate some expired cheese last night so if they come into the bathroom, they need to bring a hazmat suit. Works every time.)

Light your incense as you normally would. Place a couple of drops on the Manifest That Shit Oil on your tealight, then light that bitch up. Place the incense and the candle right next to each other on your work space, and place your journal right in front.

Open the journal to its first page. On this page, write a manifestation incantation that includes a protection from wandering eyes (malicious or not). I've provided an example, but feel free to alter it to fit you better. Pro tip: I like to translate my incantations (journal-specific ones anyway) into Latin. In my head, whoever picks up my journal and reads the first page will be automatically creeped out and put it down anyway.

Write: *"Earth and space, universe surrounds. Hear my manifestations as I write them out. Stop all wandering eyes for whom this is not meant. And if they succeed, everything they read they will forget. Bless this journal and everything inside because it is an extension of what is in my mind. May all negative thoughts and energy be deterred; send those elsewhere in the world. I am worthy of my hopes and dreams; I am also worthy of success and peace. As it is said, so it is done. The universe and I are as one."*

Flip to the last page. It's time for your gratitude incantation. This will thank the universe, gods, goddesses, ancestors, spirit guides, or whomever the fuck you pray to for these things.

Write: *Thank you, thank you from the bottom of my heart for assisting me on this journey from end to start. The gifts I receive are a blessing and sacred to me; thank you for everything you've given times three. From money to love, protection to hope; I give you all my gratitude because you deserve it the most. May this prayer be an offering to keep me in your grace regardless of what comes in the following days. As it is said, so it is done. The universe and I are as one."*

Again, feel free to edit as needed. It doesn't even need to rhyme; I've just been on a streak.

Next—and hear me out—pick your journal up and kiss it. Yeah, I know, its fucking weird. Just trust me, okay? Damn.

Keep your journal on your nightstand overnight with the piece of clear quartz placed right on top. The next day (or the next time you have the will to live), you can start decorating.

Use stickers, paint pens, glitter, cutouts—anything that calls to you. The journal should be decorated in a way that represents you and your personality.

Once you're satisfied with the way your journal looks, read the first page incantation and the last page incantation once. Your journal is now ready to use whenever the fuck you want. (Keep it on your nightstand in the meantime.)

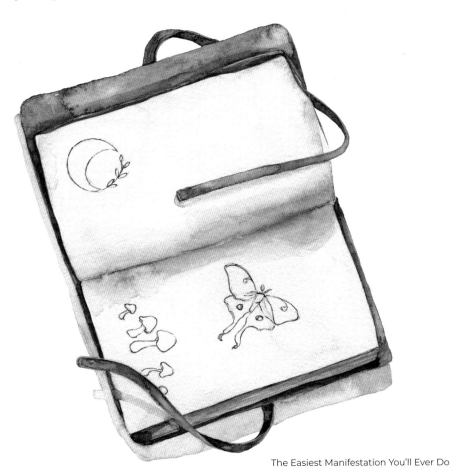

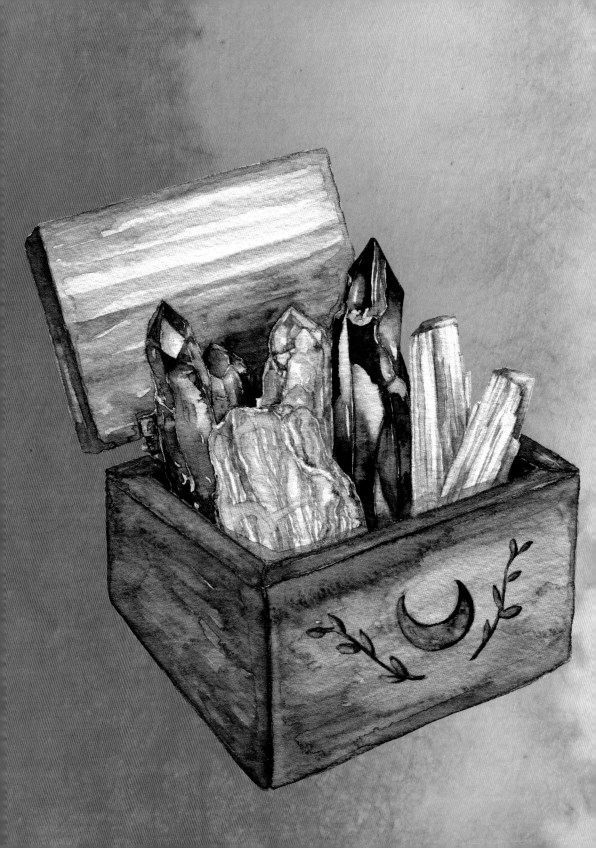

MANIFESTATION CRYSTAL BOX

THIS MANIFESTATION BOX is an easy way to simply throw your manifestations in and let them grow on their own. It's ideal for long-term manifestations and wishes. The box itself can be literally any box you like, but make sure you actually like it. Glass, wood, resin, cardboard, plastic, cement, ceramic—ANY KIND (I cannot stress this enough). Make sure it's big enough to hold your crystals along with any spell papers you want to throw in periodically.

A box

Sea salt

Amethyst

Moonstone

Blue lace agate

Obsidian

Selenite

Lunar Manifestation Herb Blend (see page 41)

Cover the bottom of your box completely with the salt. If you don't have sea salt, table salt will work just fine.

Add in each crystal, one by one, while repeating this chant: *"Crystals, moon, and the universe above, grant me my wishes as they may come. Guide me with your energy to help them come true, as you move through me and I move through you."*

Next, take a pinch of your herb blend and sprinkle, sprinkle, bitch. No, literally, sprinkle it all over everything. Say: *"Herbs and flowers, plants and roots, ground my energy and keep it in tune."*

Close your box, and hold it in your hands. Say: *"Wish box, dream box, manifest for me. Lunar energies guide me like you do the sea. All my dreams come true, so mote it be."*

Keep your box on your altar and add in your wishes/manifestations as they come to you. Once the box is filled, go through your papers, and see which ones came true. Take those out and burn them. Leave the rest inside until they're done. Finish the spell off with a gratitude ritual for everything the box helped you manifest.

NEW MOON, FULL MOON BATH SALTS

THE FOLLOWING TWO recipes are for bath salts that correspond to the new and full phases of the moon. If you don't like baths, relax. I don't either, babe. There are a few ways you can use these salts, but whichever way you choose, make sure that you're making them and using them during the correct phase of the moon. The time of day doesn't matter as long as the moon phase is correct. That's when the manifestation energy will be at its most powerful.

These salts are designed to be used in a larger bathing ritual that you can and should customize according to your own preferences. Lighting candles, surrounding the tub in crystals, and setting the mood with music are all great things to add to your bath to make your experience better. You can bring your manifestation journal in the tub with you and write while soaking to amplify your intentions.

If you don't have access to a bathtub or just hate baths, like me, I have a few suggestions for you. The first is my go-to: place the salts in a sachet and tie them around your showerhead. This is my favorite method because I shower in Satan-approved water temperatures and the steam releases all the aromas and basically acts as an "activation" for the spell. You could also use the salts as a foot soak instead of a full body soak. Or you can add about 2 ounces (59 ml) more olive oil to the mix and make it into a scrub. (Just don't use it on your face because salt is a pretty harsh exfoliant. Using it on your legs before shaving would be perfect.)

The New Moon Bath Salts will help with new beginnings and fresh starts, which is what we need when we're manifesting throughout the lunar month. The Full Moon Bath Salts, on the other hand, are great for success, accomplishment, and fertility (not babies fertility, more like life fertility). They will give you that final push you need to achieve your goal for the month. The ingredients are different, but the process is similar. If a full-on bathing ritual sounds like a lot of time or energy, don't worry. You don't need to take an hour-long bath, y'all. Ten to fifteen minutes will do just fine.

NEW MOON SALTS

6 parts pink salt

1 part sandalwood bark

1 part willow bark

1 part cherry bark

1 part orris root

½ ounce (15 ml) olive oil

20 to 30 drops of gardenia or patchouli essential oil

Bay leaves (one per manifestation goal)

2-ounce (59-ml) jar

First, combine your salt and herbs in a bowl. You'll set your intentions with the incantation at the end of this spell, so you don't have to do it now but you're more than welcome to. Add in your olive oil next, and finish with your essential oils. Do not mix yet.

Next, write down your goals for the upcoming lunar cycle on your bay leaves—one goal per leaf. You can summarize each goal into one word or create a sigil for this. Crush the bay leaves and add them to your bowl.

As you mix everything together, stir clockwise to send the wishes out into the universe. Recite the following affirmation when doing this part: *"I am confident in the moon as I am in myself. Bring me my wishes, free from fear and doubt; with this new beginning, we start from the ground."*

Store your salts in your jar. Your salts will be good to use for up to a month.

FULL MOON SALTS

6 parts black salt (see page 44)

1 part rose petals

1 part jasmine

1 part passionflower

1 part lemon balm

½ ounces (15 ml) olive oil

20 to 30 drops of rose or jasmine essential oil

2-ounce (59-ml) jar

Combine your salt and herbs in your bowl first, then add in your olive oil and finish with your essential oils. Stir the mixture counterclockwise while reciting the following affirmation to send it out into the universe.

"Lunar goddess, high as you are, let this petition reach that far. It's time for my goals to come to fruition. Give me one last burst of energy to boost my final mission."

Store the salts in a 2-ounce (59-ml) jar. Your salts will be good to use for up to a month.

Note: Leave out the essential oils if you have sensitive skin; the herbs alone do a wonderful job in this spell.

FULL MOON RELEASE
MILK RECIPE

MOON MILK IS basically tea, usually sweet, brewed with milk instead of water. The full moon isn't only outstanding for manifestation, it's perfect for releasing all things that no longer serve you to make room for your new goals and dreams. There are no substitutions in this tea, so stick with the recipe on this one, babe. Otherwise, it might not taste so good.

1 purple candle

1 tablespoon rose petals

1 tablespoon (15 ml) chamomile

1 teaspoon (5 ml) passionflower

1 teaspoon (5 ml) yarrow

Tea strainer

8 ounces (237 ml) milk of your choice

Tea cup

A dash vanilla extract

A pinch of nutmeg

Sugar or honey, to taste

A pinch of cinnamon

Paper and pen

Fireproof bowl

Light your candle before making your tea.

Combine rose, chamomile, passionflower, and yarrow in a tea strainer. Heat up your milk (boil it on the stove or in the microwave—just make sure it's hot as fuck) and pour it into your tea cup. Steep your tea in the milk for 2 to 3 minutes.

Once you've finished steeping, add in vanilla, nutmeg, sugar or honey, and cinnamon. Go sparingly with these ingredients. You can always add, but you can never take it away once it's in there.

Stir your tea counterclockwise three times.

Sip your tea for a minute, and let the energies enter your body.

Once you've drunk about half the tea, grab your paper and write down everything you want to release from your life: people who no longer serve you, spaces you no longer want to be in, habits you want to break. Whatever you want gone, write it down.

When you're finished writing, fold your paper up and burn it by holding it over your lit purple candle and dropping it into a firesafe bowl to finish burning. If fire is scary for you, burn a corner instead.

Finish your tea, blow out your candle, and discard your ashes down the drain. If you only burned a corner, discard the paper outside of your home.

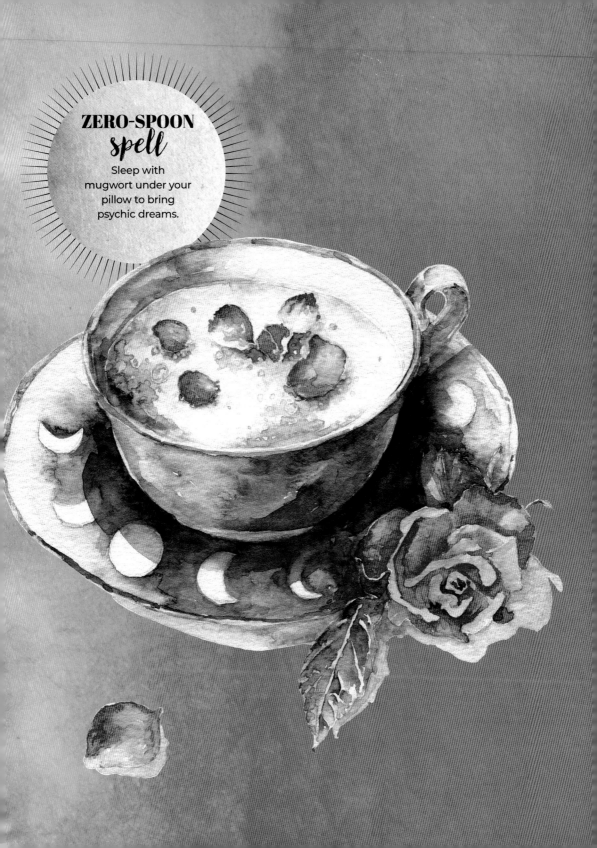

ZERO-SPOON
spell

Sleep with mugwort under your pillow to bring psychic dreams.

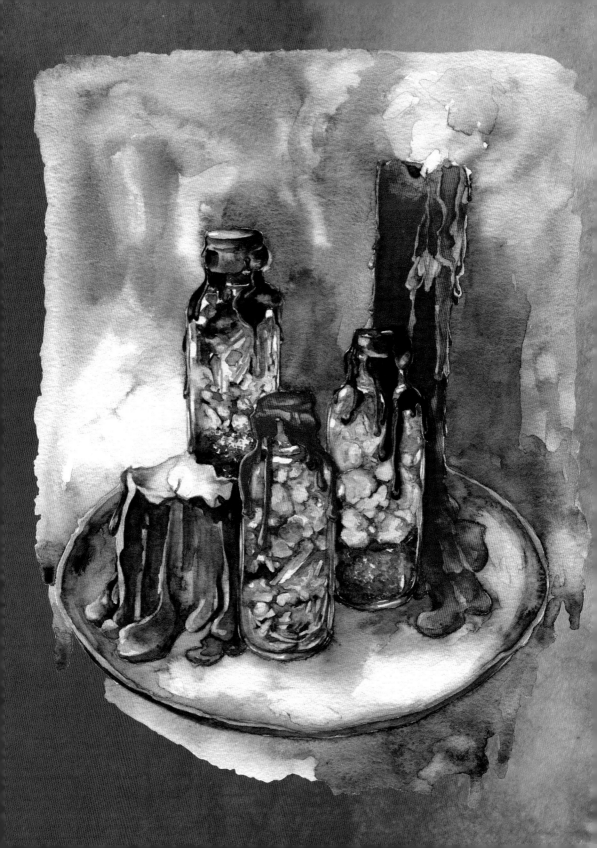

3

SPELLS FOR
protection
+
banishing

THIS IS MY FAVORITE CHAPTER, Y'ALL.

Whether you're a beginner or a fully seasoned witch, protection will be the most important type of witchcraft you do. This goes double if you're someone who struggles on the reg with your mental, physical, or emotional health. Protection spells help with so many things. They can offer spiritual and psychic protection against other witches or negative entities; physical protection for children, pets, homes, and yourself; and emotional protection for empaths who have to fight off energy vampires as if they're actually sucking your blood.

Protection spells don't only protect against intentional or unintentional magical attacks; they can protect from environmental negativity, spirits who are off their fucking rockers, and run-of-the-mill shit vibes.

There are a few different kinds of protection we can use:

WARDING

Basically, this builds an invisible bubble around whatever you're trying to protect. Warding won't send bad energy in another direction but will disintegrate whatever shit comes your way. This is also called *banishing*.

REFLECTIONS

This kind of spellwork is similar to warding in the sense that it energetically places a "mirror" in front of you. However, with reflections, if and when another practitioner sends something nasty your way, your mirror makes it automatically fall back on them. Think of it like an Uno reverse card. This is also called *reversal*.

CONCEALMENT

Concealment spells hide you or whatever you're protecting, because, bitch, if they can't find you, they can't send you some trash-ass hex. Concealment spells can also include the use of decoys (don't worry, we'll get into that later in this chapter).

DEFENSIVE PROTECTION

Our last type of protection will stop the negative shit, reverse the original spell/hex/jinx/curse, AND add on a little extra spice on its way back. For these, I suggest adding a loophole. Something along the lines of, "I hope they step on Legos at least three times a day until they learn to be a better person." Adding a loophole gives the other person, place, or thing a way to get out of your defensive spell by changing their behavior to do something society doesn't frown upon.

Throughout this chapter, I'll show you the easy way to do each one of these types of protections, so you are better equipped to safeguard your mind, body, heart, and soul. This is especially important when you're feeling stressed, ill, or low energy. When you're in those states, it super easy for other people to intentionally or unintentionally send negative energy your way or even steal the little bit of energy you have. Now mind you, if you're battling a wildly strong witch, you might have to use some more heavy-duty curses. However, that's more than likely not the case.

Before I move on to the good shit, remember to cleanse before protecting! Visit page 23 to see some ways to cleanse and choose whatever method works best for you.

> What's the difference between a jinx, a curse, and a hex? A jinx is a small inconvenience. Think, "I hope all the batteries in your house die and you have no replacements." A hex is meant to harm the target with no long-lasting side effects, while a curse is meant to cause long-lasting harm to your target.

MATERIALS AND CORRESPONDENCES FOR LAZY WITCH
protection spells

In this chapter, we'll use correspondences for protection, banishing, and reversal. The table below lists the complete correspondences for each of these intentions.

CORRESPONDENCES FOR PROTECTION, BANISHING, AND REVERSAL SPELLS

	Protection	Banishing	Reversal
Moon Phase	Full, waning, waxing	Waning	Waning
Zodiac	Cancer, Taurus	Capricorn	Capricorn
Day of the Week	Monday, Saturday, Sunday	Saturday	Saturday
Colors	Black, blue, brown, green, purple, red	Black, green, purple	Black, orange, red
Tarot Card	The Empress	The High Priestess	The Hanged Man
Herbs, Plants, and Flowers	Birch, cedar, elderberries, hawthorn, willow, angelica, basil, chrysanthemum, comfrey, lavender, pennyroyal, thyme, thistle, cinnamon, clove, mandrake, sandalwood	Elderberry, juniper, pine, angelica, basil, comfrey, clove, peppermint, rue, St. John's wort, vervain, frankincense, horehound, mandrake, mullein, nettle, patchouli	Mugwort, rose, pine needle, galangal root, cedar, rue, basil, pennyroyal, clove, thistle, mandrake, agrimony, angelica, ginger, nutmeg, mullein
Crystals and Gemstones	Amethyst, tiger's eye, red jasper, jet, obsidian, tourmaline, smoky quartz, pyrite, garnet, hematite	Aquamarine, bloodstone, red jasper, rhodonite, hematite, clear quartz, smoky quartz, tourmaline	Carnelian, red jasper, garnet, onyx, obsidian, smoky quartz, tourmaline

Here are the ingredients we'll use in this chapter

with their substitutions, so you don't lose your shit trying to find everything.

PLANTS, HERBS, AND FLOWERS

Ingredient	Substitution
Agrimony	Hyssop
Angelica	Burdock
Basil	Rosemary
Bay leaf	No substitute
Black salt	Sea Salt
Burdock	Angelica
Chai	Vanilla black tea
Cinnamon sticks	Whole clove
Comfrey	Galangal root
Elderberry	Juniper berry
Frankincense	Myrrh
Galangal root	Comfrey
Hyssop	Agrimony
Juniper berry	Elderberry
Lavender	Chamomile
Mullein	Mugwort
Myrrh	Frankincense

Ingredient	Substitution
Nettle	Pine needle
Pine needle	Nettle
Red chili pepper	Cayanne pepper
Rose	Chrysanthemum
Rosemary	Basil
Sea Salt	Table salt
St. John's wort	Yarrow
Vervain	Rue

CRYSTALS AND GEMSTONES

Ingredient	Substitution
Black tourmaline	Obsidian
Clear quartz	No substitute
Obsidian	Onyx
Red jasper	Carnelian
Smoky quartz	Clear quartz
Tiger's eye	Hematite

OTHER SHIT

Ingredient	Substitution
Moon water	Purified water
Nails	Thorns
Olive oil	Castor oil
Rubbing alcohol	No substitute
Thorns	Nails
Witch hazel (liquid)	No substitute

BASIC SIGILS, OILS, TEALIGHTS, AND BLENDS FOR *protection*

TWO-INGREDIENT TEALIGHTS FOR PROTECTION

NOTHING COULD BE easier than a simple tealight spell. The process is the same for all intentions, only the herbs and crystals change.

Tealight

Herbs and Crystals

- **Protection:** elderberry and obsidian chips
- **Warding:** pine needle and tourmaline chips
- **Banishing:** angelica and smoky quartz chips

First, set your intentions. Light the candle, and let the wax melt a bit. Blow out when you have a melty surface.

Sprinkle your herbs and crystal chips on top of the melted wax, being careful and cautious NOT to let the herb near the flame.

Save the candle for later or light it right away, and that's it!

PROTECTION SIGILS

FOR QUICK-AND-EASY protection work, create sigils (see page 29) for the following intentions and use as directed.

- Draw "PROTECTION" on the inside of your front door with a dragon's blood essential oil.
- Write "BITCH BE GONE" in the air with your finger behind the person you want to leave you the fuck alone.
- Draw "WARDING" in the dirt with a stick in your front yard to ward your home.

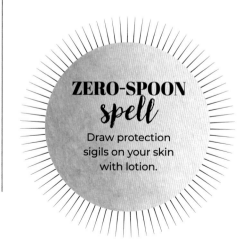

ZERO-SPOON *spell*

Draw protection sigils on your skin with lotion.

BITCH BE GONE OIL

OUR BITCH BE GONE oil will be used throughout this chapter. This oil gives off banishing, reversal, warding, and general protection vibes, making it super versatile. The only reason I gave these two spoons instead of one is for the simple fact that it requires patience. You'll see.

Agrimony

Burdock

Mullein

Rosemary

Obsidian chips

2-ounce (59-ml) dropper bottle

Olive oil (or castor oil)

Black salt (see page 44)

The patience of a monk teaching kindergarteners

Fragrance or essential oil of your choice (optional)

Start by adding your herbs one at a time to your dropper bottle, telling each one as you add it why the fuck you're gathered here today. Add your herb, say the chant. Super easy.

"Agrimony, banish anything thrown my way.
Burdock, send the negative vibes back to the darkest
depths of hell.
Mullein, create an invisibility shield so the shit vibes can't
even find me.
Rosemary, defend against any spirits that are here to bring
harmful energy."

Next, add your obsidian chips to the dropper bottle and recite the following chant: *"Protect me from everything and anything that tries to enter the space with the intent to cause harm. If I cannot see it, sound the alarm. So it is said, so it shall be."*

Next, fill the bottle with your olive oil. I recommend filling it up once, then poking the herbs in the bottle with a stick or long probe. This will allow the oil to fill in all the spots it couldn't. Then add more oil to actually fill it completely. Remember to leave space for the dropper. Once it's filled completely, seal the bottle.

Now comes the patience that I mentioned earlier. You need to leave the dropper OUTSIDE for two to three days. We want both lunar and solar energy to charge this one, because why wouldn't we want two of the most powerful celestial bodies working together for this oil?

Once your oil is charged, you can add your essential or fragrance oil, if using. Make sure the scent generally goes with the protection vibes. (Floral scents protect, too.)

And you're done! Use this oil to anoint yourself, your tools, and your crystals.

PROTECTION AND WARDING HERB BLEND

I HAD TO add an easy herb blend for y'all to have as a backup in case you need to do protection work one day and can't find the time, energy, or patience to do a whole spell from scratch. This one will also be used in multiple spells throughout the chapter.

Rosemary

Mullein

Agrimony

Angelica

Burdock

Black salt (see page 44)

Frankincense

Basil

A storing container

1 piece of clear quartz

Add the herbs to a bowl one at a time in whatever order you like. Repeat the following incantation as you place each different herb in the bowl.

"I am always protected, safe, and secure. I have faith that the universe is constantly keeping an eye on me, guiding me in a divine manner, and shielding me from harm. My light shield prevents negative influences and energies from getting through. An energy of love and protection envelops me, keeping me safe and secure. I am appreciative of this defense and have faith that it will always be there for me. I'm grateful to the universe for keeping me secure."

Mix your herbs together with your hands, and transfer them into your container of choice.

Place your clear quartz in the container on top of your herbs.

This blend will last eight to twelve months, making it so perfect for lazy spells. You can use it for sprays, baths, spell bags, jars, and incense, and to charge items on—pretty much anything you can think of. But for the love of everything holy and unholy, DO NOT EAT IT. The frankincense and black salt make that a big, fat no-no.

LAZY WITCH SPELLS AND RITUALS FOR
protection, banishing + reversal

THE EASIEST FUCKING PROTECTION SPELL

I'M BEING VERY literal with the name of this spell. Minimum effort, minimum ingredients, maximum protection.

Bay leaf

Pen

Tealight candle

Black salt (see page 44)

Start by drawing a sigil for PROTECTION on your bay leaf with your pen. (See page 29 for how to make a sigil.)

Carefully, lift the tealight out of its metal cup. You can usually gently pull the wick up while pulling the cup in the opposite direction. If it's not being cooperative, put it on its side and roll it across a flat surface to loosen the wax.

Crush your bay leaf into the empty cup. add a pinch of black salt, and place your tealight back into its rightful spot.

Light your candle, and you're done. See? So easy. You can burn it all at once or in five-minute intervals.

Discard the finished tealight outside of the home.

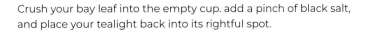
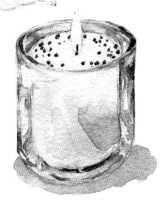

FOUR CORNER HOME PROTECTION CHARM BAGS

YOUR HOME IS the most sacred space you'll ever have, so it needs to be well-protected. The four corners of your home correspond to the points on a compass: north, south, east, and west. The north represents earth—abundance, healing, growth, wealth, and health. The east represents air—communication, life, family, community, and new beginnings. The south represents fire—creativity, passion, love, and warmth. The west represents water—emotions, balance, compassion, imagination, and psychic ability. In this spell, we'll be protecting each corner with a custom spell bag. If you share a space with other humans and only want to protect your room, you can absolutely do that instead.

Black salt

Sea salt

Pink salt

Angelica

Burdock root

Rosemary

4 small black fabric pouches

2 obsidian tumbles

1 smoky quartz (point or tumble)

1 tourmaline chunk

Combine all of the herbs and salts in a bowl in the following order: black salt, sea salt, pink salt, angelica, burdock, and rosemary.

As you add in your herbs, repeat the following affirmation. By the time you're done adding, you should have recited this at least six times.

"I am protected. I am safe. I am shielded. I am surrounded by positive energy and that is the only energy allowed in this space."

Divide the contents of the bowl between your four pouches.

Add an obsidian tumble to two of the pouches. These pouches are for your east and west corners. Take your pouches to their respective corners, and leave them there. (You can leave them on the floor or hang them on the wall.)

Add your smoky quartz to one of the remaining pouches. Place the pouch in the north corner.

Add your tourmaline to the last pouch. Place it in the south corner.

Once all your pouches have found their new homes, repeat the affirmation from above three times. You're done! You can recharge your pouches once a month on the full moon by literally just leaving them outside to soak up all the vibes.

RITUAL PROTECTION NECKLACE

WHETHER YOU'RE DOING a full-scale ritual or a simple candle spell, protection is always important. This "spell jar necklace" makes it super easy to protect yourself during your spellwork journey. The key to this, since it'll be used during ritual, is to not overprotect. When you overprotect, you not only block energy from getting into your sacred space, but you also potentially block it from leaving your space, which basically makes the spell invalid. Balance, babe, balance.

For this spell, a small spell jar (5 to 10 ml) works best. You can often find small jar charms in craft stores that already have an eyelet and jump ring attached—this will make the spell even less work. If you happen to find one, perfect, but we're going to go through the spell as if you hadn't. This will only affect the last part. Finding the premade jar turns this into a one-spoon spell.

Black salt (see page 44)

Agrimony

Rosemary

Obsidian chips

1 small spell jar with cork (5- to 10-ml jars work best for this one)

JAR CHARM MATERIALS (if creating your own):

1 jewelry-size screw eyelet

1 jump ring

1 necklace string

Jewelry-making pliers

Add the ingredients to the spell jar one at a time in the following order: black salt, agrimony, rosemary, obsidian chips. As you add each one, say: *"Shield my space from all negativities that could be headed my way. Protect me while I practice and keep that shit away. This necklace is my light, it surrounds me with all its might. May my magic make it out into the universe, but let nothing come inside."*

Place the cork in the jar, and push it in as far as you can. You don't want it to fall out randomly because that would not be cute.

Screw your eyelet into the cork. Breathe, take your time. It's tiny, and it's annoying. Once the eyelet is secure, open the jump ring. Thread it through the eyelet hole and close it. Thread your necklace string through the jump ring, and you're done!

Keep your ritual protection necklace on your altar for easy access during spells. Repeat the incantation from earlier to activate it before every use.

SEAL YOUR SPACE

THIS SPELL WILL seal in your cleansing and protective spellwork so nothing but good energy can make its way into your space. Don't worry, you don't need to do this spell on the exact same day as you do a protection spell. In fact, you don't even need to cleanse and protect on the same day either. This is lazy witchcraft and that seems like a lot. Instead, I suggest spreading this spellwork out over one week.

This spell requires a tether for your home. This can be anything that represents your home, even just a piece of paper with your address.

White candle	Light your candle and set it right next to your envelope.
1 envelope	
Angelica	Draw a "SEAL MY SPACE" sigil (see page 29) on the outside of the envelope flap.
Rosemary	
Pine needle	Flip it over and add your ingredients to the pouch. Start with the angelica, rosemary, and pine needle, followed by your crystals, and, last of all, your tether. Recite the following chant as you add in your ingredients: *"This space is mine, by will and divine. May all the energy here be healed and so it is by magic sealed."*
Smoky quartz chips	
Clear quartz chips	
Home tether	
Bay leaf	Seal the envelope like you would normally (yes, bitch, with your tongue) and then pour a tiny bit of candle wax on it to seal it even better.

Light your bay leaf with your candle and let it burn for about 3 seconds. Blow it out and pass your envelope through the smoke coming off of your bay leaf.

Keep the envelope in a safe place (literally anywhere you want in your home) until it's time to do your cleanse and protect spells again. At that time, open your envelope, remove your crystals, and discard the rest outside of your home. Then simply repeat this spell.

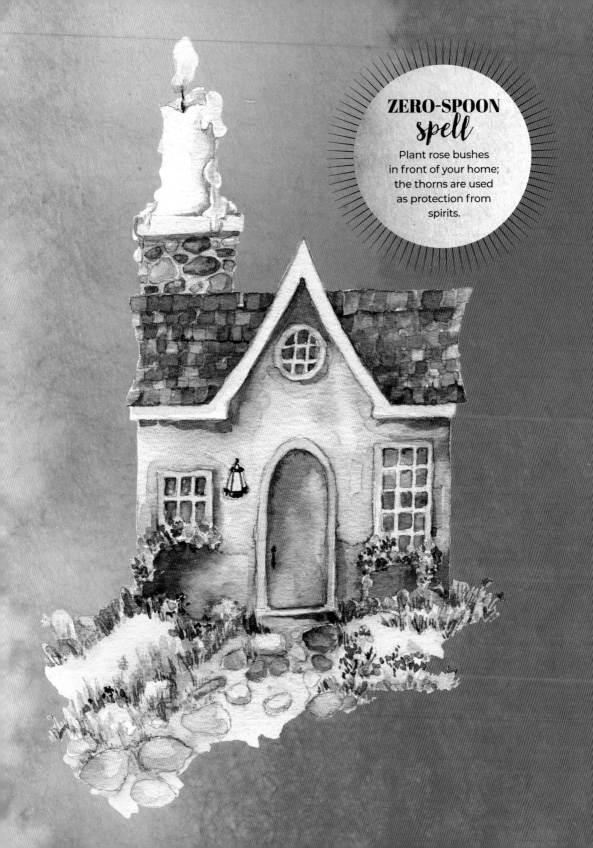

ZERO-SPOON
spell

Plant rose bushes
in front of your home;
the thorns are used
as protection from
spirits.

PET PROTECTION CANDLE SPELL

OUR PETS ARE our best friends. They're with us through the good, the bad, and the mental breakdowns at 3 am because we remembered something embarrassing we did five years ago. Did you know that our pets basically absorb energy from us? We don't realize it, they don't realize it, but it's absolutely a thing. This spell cleanses all the negativity the little ones have absorbed and adds a protective shield around them.

This spell makes use of a tether. A tether is basically an item or object that represents the subject. In this case, the subject is your pet. You can use some of their hair, which should be easy if they shed like their lives depend on it. Or you can grab a small paper and create a sigil based on your pet's name. (See page 29 for more on sigils.)

Carving tool

White chime candle

Bitch Be Gone Oil (see page 63)

Lighter

Bowl or chime candle holder

Basil

Hyssop

Comfrey

Salt (any kind)

Tiger's eye tumble

Obsidian tumble

Smoky quartz

Tether

Moon water

Start by carving a "PET PROTECTION" sigil into your candle. If your brain isn't braining, go ahead and just write the actual words.

Rub a few drops of your Bitch Be Gone Oil all over your candle. (Stay away from the wick and the bottom of the candle, which we're about to melt, or you'll end up with the biggest flame of your life.)

Take a lighter and melt the bottom of your candle just a bit. Stick it to the inside of your bowl, right in the middle. If you have a chime candle holder, you can use that instead.

Next, add your herbs to the bowl, sprinkling them right around the candle. The order isn't important here; however, your intention is, so all you're going to do is repeat this phrase:

"(Insert pet's name here) is protected. (Insert pet's name here) is shielded. (Insert pet's name here) will have no harm come their way."

Next, in no particular order, place your crystals inside the bowl around the candle. Just do what feels nice to you.

Last, add your tether. Sprinkle it inside your bowl. If you used a bay leaf or paper to create a sigil, rip it up before tossing it in.

Now, activate the spell with the moon water. Slowly pour your water into the bowl. You don't want to fill it all the way up—just enough so that the herbs float. As you pour, repeat the following chant three times:

"Protect this creature from harm, keep them safe in my arms."

Let the candle burn all the way down. When the spell is done, discard the contents outside of your home. Repeat every time you redo your own protections.

TAKE THIS AS A WARNING SPELL

ISN'T IT SO fucking annoying when someone won't leave you the fuck alone? They keep sending you negative energy and just won't stop? This is the spell you do before doing a full-on reversal spell. It's a warning to the person to stop fucking around. This can also be used on people who talk bad about you, bother you or your family, or are generally just not getting the hint that they're a terrible person. (Note that the chant reads like a threat but is just meant to scare, not to harm. Think of it as a baby jinx.)

Bitch Be Gone Oil (see page 63)

1 black candle

1 blue candle

Rub a few drops of the Bitch Be Gone oil onto your candles, avoiding the wicks. Set the candles up about 1 inch apart, wash your hands, and light the candles.

Whisper the following into the flames:

"My blood turns black; my flesh turns blue. I will curse you if you force me to. If you mess with a witch, you'll get burned like a bitch. With harm to none nor returned to me, see yourself with open eyes, so mote it be."

End the spell by blowing out your candles. You can reuse the candles or throw them out—that's up to you!

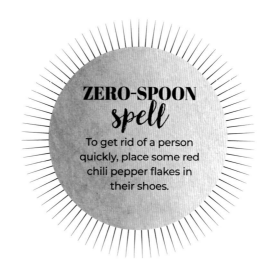

ZERO-SPOON *spell*

To get rid of a person quickly, place some red chili pepper flakes in their shoes.

"STAY THE FUCK AWAY FROM ME" SPELL JAR CHARM

DESIGNED SPECIFICALLY TO keep people or things the fuck away from you, this defensive protection spell creates a shield of energy around you that absorbs all the hits that are sent your way.

Small jar with cork

Black salt

Basil

Mullein leaf

Burdock

Obsidian chips

Red jasper chips

1 black candle

1 red candle

Evil eye charm with string (optional)

3 small cinnamon sticks (you can always break a big one into three pieces)

For this spell, we'll give each ingredient its own affirmation. Start with the black salt. As you pour it into your jar, say: *"I am protected."* Add the basil next and say: *"I am under divine protection."* Next, add the mullein leaf: *"I am safe from negative and toxic energy."* Next the burdock root: *"I am strong and grounded."* Last, add the chips. Add the obsidian first and say: *"I only allow positive vibes in my space."* Then, add the red jasper and say: *"No harm will come my way."*

Cork your jar and light your candles. You'll use the melting wax from the candles to seal your jar. If you want to add an evil eye charm, tie that around your jar before lighting the candles.

Once the candles are lit, use them to seal the entire cork with wax. Ideally, you can do it at the same time (red and black at once). If not, start by hover the black candle over one half of the cork while letting the wax drip directly onto the cork; then grab your red candle and do the same thing to finish the other side.

When that's all in there, finish by stabbing in your cinnamon stick pieces. I mean actual stabbing; we need that metaphorical energy. Say: *"And anyone who tries to cross this line, may karma take."*

Ideally, you'd carry your jar with you at all times, either in a purse or backpack. However, I am fully aware that not all of us can do that shit. I don't even like purses. If that's you, keep it by your front door or in your bedroom.

You can recharge the jar in the moonlight every few weeks or you can disassemble and remake it. Both methods have the same effect.

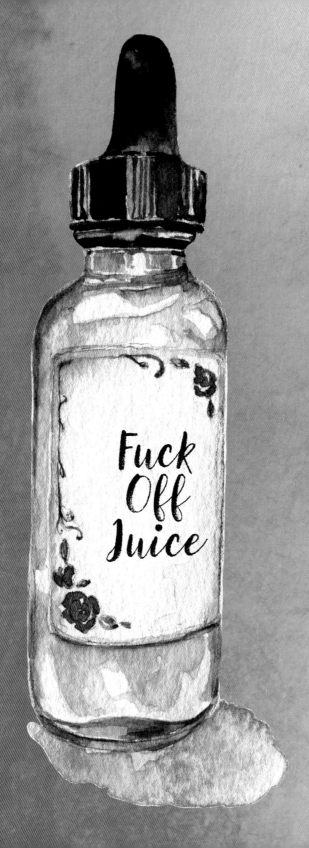

FUCK OFF JUICE

BEFORE I EVEN START, DO NOT DRINK THIS. I know I called it juice. It's a figure of speech. Don't ingest this. It'll probably taste gross anyway. This Fuck Off Juice is going to make everyone and everything you don't want around you fuck off. Think banishing spell meets protection spell. It eliminates the person, place, or thing and also protects you from letting that energy back into your space.

1-ounce (29-ml) dropper bottle

Angelica

Galangal root

Comfrey

Mullein

Elderberry

St. John's wort

Red chili pepper flakes

Sea salt

Tiger's eye tumble

Moon water (see page 19) or collected storm water

Rubbing alcohol

All the ingredients go directly into the bottle. As you add them, tell each herb why the fuck they're there:

"Angelica, banish this bitch.
Galangal, give me the damn authority to banish this bitch.
Comfrey, let me control the outcome of this situation.
Mullein, if they don't leave, send darkness their way.
Elderberry, reflect any negativity they try and leave behind.
St. John's wort, defend me against any retaliation.
Red chili pepper, make it sting a little bit so they move
*   their ass faster.*
Salt, blend my ingredients together and activate them."

Add the tiger's eye last. This will be the final "nail in the coffin," since tiger's eye is great for karma spells. Say: *"And with this tiger's eye, their karma will match their energy."*

Fill the bottle all the way with about 9 parts water and 1 part rubbing alcohol. Shake super well and keep it in a cool, dark place for at least three days before using.

To use it, put a few drops on your target's shoes. If you can't get close, find something that represents them, like a piece of clothing or a paper with personal details about them, and put your drops on those instead. They should, ideally, fuck all the way off until they have no more fucks to off.

CURSE REMOVAL WITH HEKATE

THIS INCENSE BLEND calls on Hekate, the goddess of witchcraft, to assist in removing any curse, hex, or jinx that may or may not have been placed on you. This recipe is for incense, but you can actually use it as you would any other herb blend. So feel free to dress a candle with it, charge some crystals or jewelry on it, etc.

Basil

Myrrh

Frankincense

Angelica

Rosemary

Mortar and pestle

Loose incense burner

Add your herbs to your mortar and pestle. As you add them, tell each one what they're doing.

"Basil to pinpoint where exactly the curse is. Myrrh to deal with the darkness. Frankincense to bind danger. Angelica to defend my space. Rosemary to cleanse and bless once all the bullshit is gone."

Grind up the mix until you have a fine powder. Place a small amount in your incense burner of choice. After lighting it, repeat the following chant thirteen times. Yes, I mean exactly thirteen. Don't be trying to cheat your way out of this one, y'all. I'm going to give you the English translation for the Latin version, so we don't accidentally summon any demons from hell or whatever.

"Hekate, Queen of Darkness, Mother of Witches. A curse upon my life has been cast. A dark cloud that just won't pass. Remove this obstacle from my path; send it back to where it was last. So mote it be."

Let your incense go out on its own. Use the ashes to create black salt (see page 44).

> No mortar and pestle? Use a coffee grinder to save time and energy; just remember that you won't be able to use it for food again without a proper, deep sanitizing cleanse.

REFLECT A HEX

YOU SEE THE title of this spell? That's literally what we're going to do here. Reflect the hex back to wherever the fuck it came from. For this spell, I'd prefer if you used a candle that's in a jar but if you only have chime or taper candles, grab a candle holder as well.

Small mirror (one that you can lay flat)	Lay your mirror flat on your work surface.
Black salt (see page 44)	Sprinkle black salt on your mirror and use your finger spread it over the glass like butter over toast. It doesn't need to be thick or perfectly even.
Paper	
Pen	Now it's time to write. If you know the name and birth date of the person who cursed you, write that down on the paper. If
1 black jar candle (any kind)	you don't know who the fuck it is, make a sigil from the words "PERSON WHO CURSED ME" (see page 29 for more on sigils).

Fold the paper one time, away from you, and place it on your mirror.

Place your candle right on top of the paper.

Light the candle and recite the following six times: *"I reflect this spell back to you, and for the trouble, we multiply it by two. All harm and ill intent is yours, of this we shall ensure. Come back again, and it'll triple. As it has been said, as it shall be."*

Let the candle burn for at least thirty minutes. Discard the salt and paper outside of your home. Cleanse your mirror and candle for reuse.

CHAI RITUAL FOR PROTECTION

THIS MINI TEA ritual is perfect for the end of the day. It will wash away all that nasty energy that might have gotten stuck to your aura, and it'll reset your protections so you can rest nice and easy.

Chai

Teacup

Brown sugar
(to taste)

Brew your chai like you normally would. Follow whatever instructions are on the packaging. Pour your tea into the cup. Add in your sugar. You don't need to add it if you don't like sweet drinks, but you'll still need to pretend you're stirring something in for this next part.

Stir your tea counterclockwise three times, repeating the following chant with each stir: *"I release all the bullshit from this entire day."*

Next, stir your tea clockwise three times, repeating the following chant with each stir: *"I bring back my protections to keep negativity away."*

Sip your tea and let the warmth fill your body.

Once you're about half way through your drink, repeat the incantation three more times: *"I release all the bullshit from this entire day while I bring back my protections to keep negativity away."*

Finish your tea, and the spell is complete.

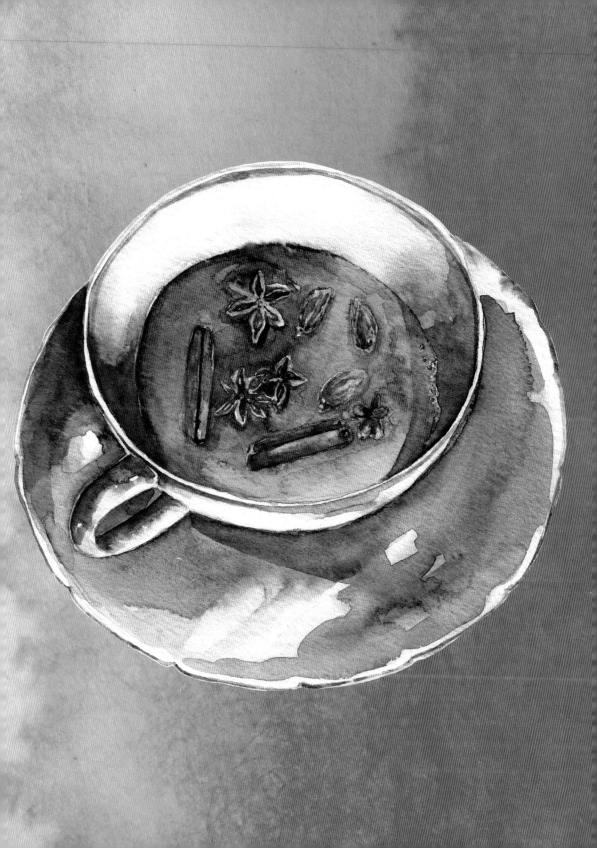

SHARP AS A THORN, TOUGH AS A NAIL: EMOTIONAL PROTECTION SPELL

THIS MINI RITUAL spell is so easy. It is a spell jar so keep that in mind while choosing your ingredients. The main ingredient here is storm water. Storms are powerful as fuck so imagine we're harnessing that pure, raw energy. Storm water is easy enough to collect; I just put a cooking pot outside and collect it that way. Just be sure to put your pot or bowl outside before the storm begins so you don't accidentally get struck by lightning, and bring it in when you're sure the storm has actually passed.

Nails (rusty nails are actually preferred)

Thorns

Nettle

Pine needle

Obsidian chips

Storm water

Rubbing alcohol

Jar with twist cap

1 black candle

Add all the solid ingredients to the jar one at a time. The order in which you add them isn't important. Before you add each one, hold the ingredient in your hands for five to ten seconds, close your eyes, and repeating the following incantation:

"Strong as lightning, thunder, and rain; all attempts to harm me will be in vain. Sharp as a thorn, tough as a nail, all who attempt to break this shield will ultimately fail."

Once all the ingredients have been added, fill about ⅛ of your jar with the rubbing alcohol. Fill the rest with storm water, but leave about ½ inch of space from the top.

Put your cap on the jar. Light your candle and seal the jar by dripping wax over top of it.

Give this spell jar a good shake whenever you're about to enter a situation where your emotions could be taken advantage of or whenever you feel in need of a bit more protection.

Recharge on your windowsill during storms.

DECOY SPELL BAG

THIS CONCEALMENT SPELL is your decoy. Someone wants to hex you? The decoy will catch it. Someone wants to spy on you? They're going to end up spying on a bag of damn herbs and crystals. Someone talks shit online about you? The bag will absorb it. The bag is you, but you are not the bag.

Strand of your hair	Place your hair in the pouch first. This will give your bag the same energy you carry.
Any small pouch	
Angelica	Add a pinch of each herb in whatever order you prefer. Once they're all in the bag, recite: *"Curiosity will kill the cat, and no amount of satisfaction can bring it back. Anyone who tries to harm me will only hurt the bag."*
Black salt (see page 44)	
Nettle	
Galangal root	Add the obsidian next and say: *"My mirror-like friend will reflect their intent right back, while cutting off the connection to my track."*
Elderberry	
Obsidian	
Clear quartz	Last, add the clear quartz and say: *"My decoy is done; we activate it now. May anyone who tries to cross me, not be allowed."*
	Keep your bag on your altar or bury it by your front door.

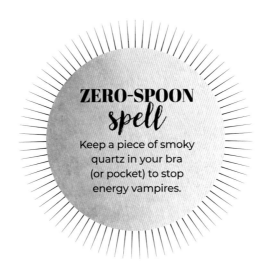

ZERO-SPOON *spell*

Keep a piece of smoky quartz in your bra (or pocket) to stop energy vampires.

STORM PROTECTION SPELL

THE EARTH IS DYING. I know it, you know it, the world knows it. Unfortunately, it looks like no one in power actually gives a shit. There are tornadoes and hurricanes, forest fires and earthquakes all in places they have never been before. This spell can't fix or reverse any of that, but it can protect your home during a storm. (Please, for the love of the gods, still do your normal storm protection. This spell is a SECOND line of defense, not a first. It isn't a replacement for storm shutters, tornado basements, or hurricane shelters.) Do this spell BEFORE the storm gets to you. If you start once it's already there, it more than likely will not work.

Lighter

1 blue candle

1 yellow candle

1 black candle

1 white candle

Heat-proof plate

Paper and pen

Dirt (from your property)

Protection and Warding Herb Blend (see page 64)

Piece of string (any color)

Use a lighter to melt the bottom of each candle and stick them onto your plate in a diamond formation. (If you have enough candle holders, you can use those instead.) As you place the candles in their appropriate places, think about the meaning of each one. Place the blue candle on the left point; this represents water and rain. Place the yellow candle on the right point; this represents thunder and lightning. Place the white candle on the top point (furthest away from you); this represents heavy winds. Place the black candle on the bottom point (closest to you); this will absorb all the damage.

Write down your address on your paper. If you prefer, you can make it into a sigil but, honestly, it's not totally necessary.

Fold the paper toward you to bring the protection into your home. Once it's small enough to fit in the middle of the candles, place it there.

Next, sprinkle the dirt directly on top of the paper. You don't need to cover the whole-ass piece; you just need a lil' pile situation.

Take a small amount of your herb blend and hold it in your hands. Recite: *"Storms and thunder, wind and rain; miss my house so here I may remain. Goddess above, moon and sun; protect me from this storm with harm to none."*

Sprinkle your herb blend all over the plate.

Before we light the candles, we need to tie our string. This is the tricky part. You need to tie it around all four candles. You can do this by tying the center of the string around one candle then looping it around the others (in clockwise or counterclockwise direction) and tying off the ends on the last candle. I usually tie the string closer to the top of the candles because fire gives me anxiety, and I'd rather get the "string burning" part of it over with quickly. Be gentle if you're not using candle holders or your candles will fall over. If this happens, just stick them back up. Not a big deal, y'all.

Once your string is secured, light your candles, babe.

Now, I'll give you two ways to finish this spell. If you're like me and fire is not your thing, blow out your candles right after they've burned down enough for the flames to light the string. The string does need to catch fire, but it does not need to be on fire for that long. Once you blow out the candles, the string should be the only thing on fire and it'll go out pretty quickly. (Pro tip: Keep sand nearby to put out any fire that gives you anxiety.)

If fire is your thing, let that bitch burn all the way down.

Discard everything AFTER THE STORM HAS PASSED. Just leave it on your altar and don't touch it until the threat has ceased to exist, babe. Then, you'll just throw it out in the trash—inside or outside, it doesn't make a difference.

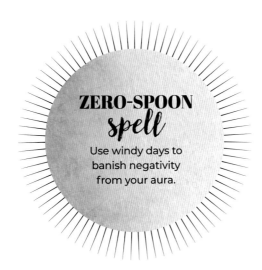

ZERO-SPOON
spell
Use windy days to banish negativity from your aura.

SLOW-RELEASE PROTECTION BOWL

SOME PROTECTION SPELLS really don't last long enough, especially for people who are always tired and don't have the energy to be repeating spells all the time. (It's me, I'm *people*.) I created this spell for anyone and everyone who forgets protection or doesn't have the energy to maintain this kind of spellwork all the time—anyone who is bedridden or my people with ADHD or other neurospicy disorders or anyone who just doesn't fucking want to do it every damn month. The ingredients are strong enough for us only having to do this twice a year, and the process is super easy.

This spell does require an offering of alcohol to the universe. You'll leave it out for an extended amount of time so hard liquor is ideal to prevent molding. Stay away from flavored liquors, wine, or beer since the sugar in them may attract flies or bugs. If you're a sober queen or king, you can switch it out for grape juice, but you may not want to leave the juice out for as long.

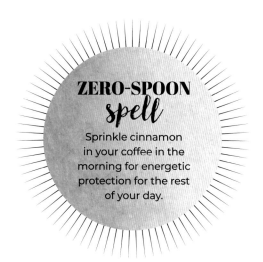

ZERO-SPOON *spell*

Sprinkle cinnamon in your coffee in the morning for energetic protection for the rest of your day.

1 pretty bowl that your roommate won't miss	Start with your herbs. They'll go into the bowl in twos. Start by adding the comfrey and angelica. While you add them, say: *"Physically protect* me."
Comfrey	
Angelica	Next, add the rose and juniper. Say: *"Emotionally protect me."*
Rose	
Juniper	Next, add the mullein leaf and galangal root. Say: *"Spiritually protect me."*
Mullein leaf	
Galangal root	Finally, add the basil and hyssop and say: *"Mentally protect me."*
Basil	
Hyssop	The last herb to go into the bowl is vervain. Vervain will supercharge the whole-ass thing. So, tell it that. As you add it, say: *"Supercharge this bitch."*
Vervain	
1 tealight (black preferred, any color is cool though)	Add the tealight to the middle of the bowl, on top of your herbs. Place your crystals around the tealight in any order.
Tourmaline	Light your candle and say: *"Moon and Sun, Goddess and God; I call upon you, over me you'll watch. Please take my offering as a gift, and let all harm be cast adrift. Protective power here now held, with this bowl and offering all harm repelled."*
Obsidian	
Smoky quartz	
Clear quartz	Let your tealight burn down all the way. Once it's done, replace it with your shot glass filled with your offering of choice.
1 shot glass	
Hard liquor of your choice	Leave the bowl on your altar and don't touch it for five to six months. It's okay if you have to change its location, but leave the contents alone, and you'll be fine.

Once your five to six months are over, discard the herbs, cleanse your crystals, and redo the exact same spell.

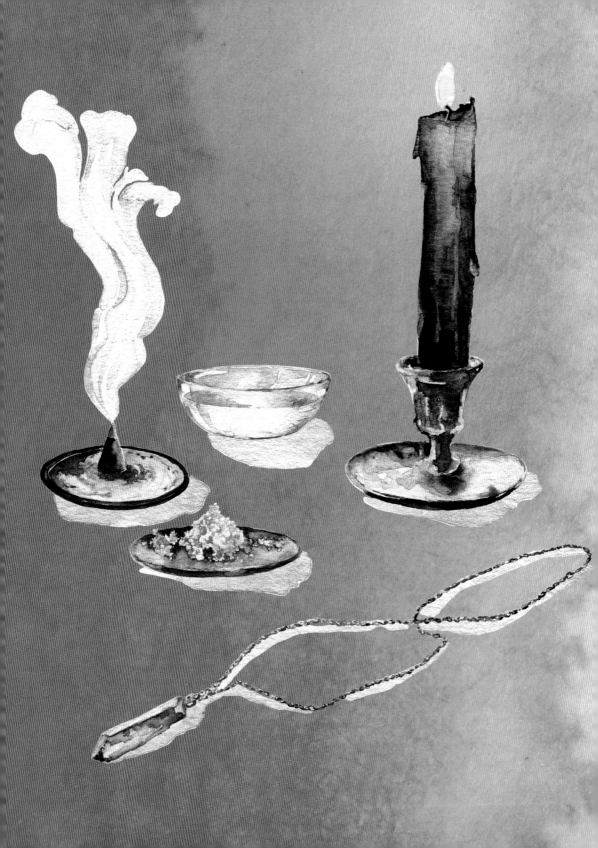

WARDING ENCHANTMENT RITUAL

FOR THIS SPELL, we'll use the four elements—earth, wind, fire, and air—to enchant any piece of jewelry you'd like to use as a ward against danger. You can also use this to enchant crystals, tools, or even your damn car keys.

Incense (choose a protective scent, see page 59)

Incense holder

1 black candle

Candle holder

Moon water

Glass bowl

Black salt (see note)

Pink salt (see note)

Sea salt (see note)

Small plate

Jewelry or item of your choice

Before you begin the spell, you need to set up your elemental stations. As you do this, try to keep them in a line formation. It'll make your life easier.

Your incense comes first; this represents air. Light it, and set it on your workspace in a holder. Next, light your candle; this represents fire. Place it next to your incense in a holder. Pour your moon water into a bowl; this represents water. Place that next to your candle. Last are the salts, which represent earth. Place the plate next to the bowl, and add in the salts. Mix them with your hands if you're using all three.

Now you can start enchanting your talisman. Start by placing your jewelry, keys, or object in the salt mixture. Leave it in there for 14 seconds. Say: *"Power of earth, protect me spiritually, emotionally and physically. So, mote it be."*

Next, dip your talisman in your water four times. Say: *"Power of water, protect me from all ill-will."*

Hold your talisman over the incense, making sure the smoke goes directly onto your item. Hold it there for 14 seconds. Say: *"Power of ai, protect me from negativity."*

Last is our fire. Pass the talisman over your candle flame a total of four times. Say: *"Power of fire, protect me from harm."*

And you're done! Your talisman is ready to use. When you feel yourself needing an extra boost of protection, just repeat this ritual. The talisman should remain charged for three to four weeks.

Note: This recipe calls for three different types of salt. If you don't have all of them, that's okay. You'll be fine with just one.

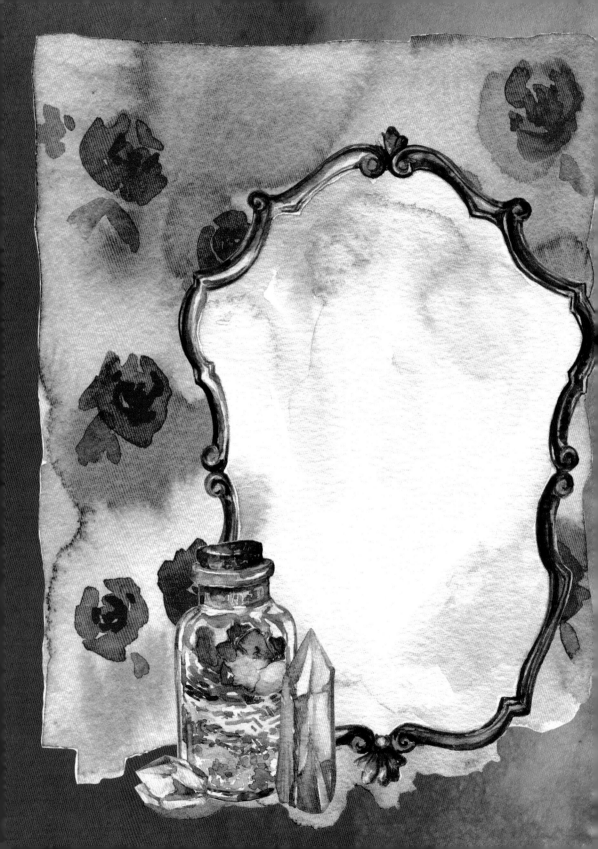

4

SPELLS FOR
healing + self-love

Like protection, this is one of my all-time favorite types of witchcraft to work with, especially when I'm feeling shitty. Shitty days are normal; stress is normal; negative thoughts are normal. We're not here to suppress or eradicate those feelings; that's not what healing and self-love spellwork is about. Instead, it's about coping with them when they do arise, adding onto our already present self-care routines, and supporting our belief in our own self-worth, even when (especially when!) it's really, really hard.

The spells in this chapter will help get rid of that little voice in the back of your head that's telling you that you're not good enough. They will instill strength, courage, and inner peace, while assisting you in your healing journey. Think of this chapter as a vitamin supplement that specifically targets your self-worth because, babe, you're worth so much. These spells are what this book is all about: easy, self-affirming magic for those days when your stress or anxiety or depression monsters are at full strength. If any of these spells make you feel even 15 percent better, my mission has been accomplished.

MATERIALS AND CORRESPONDENCES FOR LAZY WITCH
healing + self-love

The spells in this chapter will be based on a few different correspondences, mainly self-love, healing, happiness, and cleansing.

I've sprinkled in a little peace, harmony, and joy, too, but we'll cover those correspondences on a spell-by-spell basis. Before we get started, I need to say: I am not a doctor, I am not an herbalist, and this chapter is not a replacement for medication. Witchcraft is meant to enhance what's already there, which also means enhancing the properties of your medications. PLEASE see a doctor or talk to someone if your bad thoughts are leaning toward self-harm. I love you, the universe loves you, and I need you to love you, too.

CORRESPONDENCES FOR SELF-LOVE, HEALING, HAPPINESS, AND CLEANSING

	Love	Healing
Moon Phase	Full, waxing	Full
Zodiac	Cancer, Libra	Aquarius, Scorpio
Colors	Mauve, red, pink, white	Brown, gold, green, pink, white
Tarot Card	The Lovers	The Sun
Herbs, Plants, and Flowers	Apple, cherry, basil, chrysanthemum, daisy, calendula, mugwort, rose, yarrow, burdock, cardamom, cinnamon, galangal, orris, sandalwood	Birch, cedar, elderflower, willow, angelica, chamomile, lavender, lemon balm, yarrow, passionflower, skullcap, sandalwood, cinnamon, thistle
Crystals and Gemstones	Amazonite, amethyst, desert rose, garnet, malachite, rhodochrosite, rose quartz, aquamarine	Amethyst, apatite, blue lace, citrine, celestite, moonstone, moss agate, rose quartz, clear quartz, sunstone

To save you time, money, and fucking stress, I added this nice little cheat sheet of magical substitutions to help you out when you realize you're missing an ingredient.

CRYSTALS AND GEMSTONES

Ingredient	Substitution
Citrine	Carnelian
Clear quartz	No substitute
Moonstone	Fluorite
Rose quartz	Amethyst
Sunstone	Mookaite

CARRIER OILS AND ESSENTIAL OILS

Ingredient	Substitution
Coconut oil	Olive oil
Jasmine essential oil	Jasmine
Lavender essential oil	Lavender
Olive oil	Avocado oil
Rose essential oil	Rose
Sandalwood essential oil	Sandalwood

Happiness	Cleansing
Waning	Waning
No substitute	Virgo
Gold, yellow, light blue, white	Blue, lavender, purple, white
The Empress	The Sun
Cherry bark, hawthorn leaf, juniper, basil, catnip, jasmine, lilac, lily, calendula, mugwort, rose, thyme, yarrow, frankincense, patchouli	Birch, elderflower, pine needle, chamomile, dill, jasmine, lavender, passionflower, rose, vervain, yarrow, thistle, cinnamon, frankincense, sandalwood
Aquamarine, aventurine, blue lace, garnet, hematite, moonstone, moss agate, rose quartz	Amethyst, ametrine, aragonite, fluorite, obsidian, clear quartz, tourmaline, tiger's eye

PLANTS, HERBS, AND FLOWERS

Ingredient	Substitution
Calendula	Sunflower
Chamomile	Lavender
Clove	Cinnamon
Dragon's blood incense	Frankincense
Frankincense	Myrrh
Elderflower	Elderberry
Hibiscus	Orris root
Jasmine	Chrysanthemum
Lavender	Blessed thistle
Lemon balm	Lemongrass
Nettle	Skullcap
Passionflower	Chamomile
Rose petals	Dandelion
Rosehips	Hibiscus
Sandalwood	Myrrh
Skullcap	Passionflower
Yarrow	St. John's wort

OTHER SHIT

Ingredient	Substitution
Bay Leaves	Paper (for this chapter)
Cinnamon sticks	Cardamom pods
Lemon juice	Lime juice
Lemon slices	Lime slices
Orange slices	Ginger
Pink salt	Sea salt
Sea salt	Table salt
Sea shells	No substitute
Sugar	No substitute

BASIC TEALIGHTS, SIGILS, AND BLENDS FOR
healing + self-love

We'll start this chapter with some easy tealights, sigils, and oil-and-herb blends to promote good vibes on bad days.

TWO-INGREDIENT TEALIGHTS FOR HEALING AND SELF-LOVE

Tealight

Herbs and Crystal Chips:

- **Healing:** Chamomile and clear quartz
- **Self-Love:** Rose petals and rose quartz
- **Tranquility:** Elderflower and moonstone
- **Mental Health Reset:** Passionflower and rose quartz
- **Grounding:** Jasmine and clear quartz

Let the wax melt a bit. Blow out the flame when you have a melty surface. Sprinkle your herbs and crystal chips on top of the melted wax, being careful and cautious NOT to let the herb near the flame. That's it. Save it for later or use it right away.

SELF-LOVE AND HEALING SIGILS

TO EASILY BRING a little extra healing and self-love into your life, create sigils (see page 29) for the following intentions and use as directed.

- Draw "SELF-LOVE" on your bathroom mirror with a dry erase marker (dry erase markers make for easy clean-up later).
- Write "HEALING" on your journal/ diary/book of shadows.
- Add "GROUND" to the bottoms of your shoes.

SELF LOVE AND HEALING OIL

THIS OIL BLEND has multiple correspondences and will be used throughout the chapter, so I recommending you make it first so it's ready to be called into action when you need it. You can use it in peace spells and happiness spells, such as, if your home feels "angry" (you're having constant arguments, you feel on edge all the time). It can help strengthen your relationships and also takes care of imposter syndrome like a fucking champ.

The recipe is for a ½ ounce (15 ml) bottle. (If you're using a 1-ounce [29-ml] bottle, just multiply the recipe by two). I've listed five herbs that work well in this oil, but you only need three; so choose whatever is easiest for you. (Of course, you can use all five if you're feeling extra, like I usually am.)

Rose petals

Passionflower

Jasmine

Yarrow

Lavender

Rose quartz chips

1 tablespoon (12 ml) fractionated coconut oil

20 drops of rose essential oil or

20 drops of lavender essential oil

Small tray or plate

1-tablespoon (15-ml) dropper bottle

Gloves

For this oil, we need to charge our items before we do the spell. Place all your ingredients (herbs, crystal chips, and oils) on a tray or plate and leave it outside overnight. The moon will charge that bad boy and make everything extra potent. Bring everything inside the following day, and you're ready to begin.

Start by adding your herbs one at a time, until the bottle is about a third full. As you add each one, tell them why they're there.

"Rose, you're here to bring me unconditional love. Passionflower, you're here to calm me the fuck down. Jasmine, you're here to heal my emotional despair."

(And so on. You could be less dramatic with it, but what fun is that? See the correspondence table on page 90 if you need some ideas for how to communicate the correct intentions to your ingredients.)

Next, add your chips, again stating why you've brought them here: *"Rose quartz, you're here on behalf of Aphrodite to make me love myself once more."*

Next, add your essential oils. Put your gloves on right the fuck now or else those oils will stick to your skin, and you'll smell it for the entire day. Not even washing your hands will save you. You can use lavender and rose together if you'd like or just choose one. Finish the spell by filling the rest of the bottle with the coconut oil. (Remember not to overfill or your dropper will not fit in the bottle, and it will 1,000 percent overflow.)

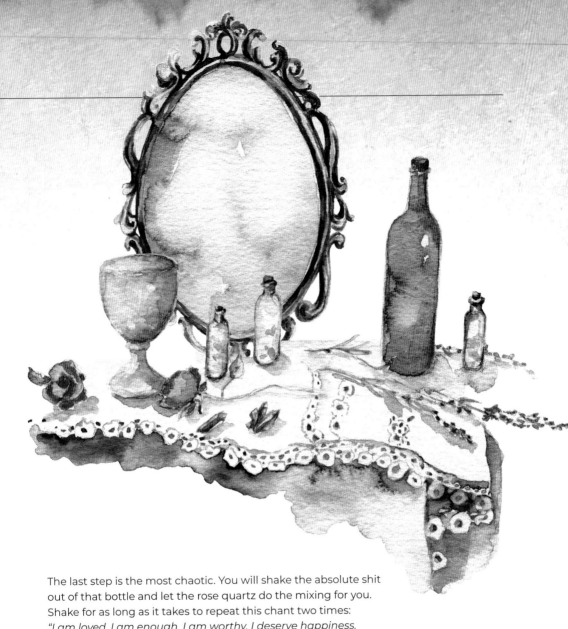

The last step is the most chaotic. You will shake the absolute shit out of that bottle and let the rose quartz do the mixing for you. Shake for as long as it takes to repeat this chant two times: *"I am loved. I am enough. I am worthy. I deserve happiness. I deserve love. I will be okay."*

Store it on your vanity or wherever you get ready for the day. Use it on your pressure points or behind your ears. Recharge by placing it in the moonlight overnight when you feel it needs a bit of a magical boost.

SELF-LOVE HERBAL MIX

HERB MIXES ARE my favorite for lazy witches. You can use them for so many things. Baths, teas, charging tools and crystals, incense, candle dressing, solid floor washes, spray bases—I could honestly go on forever. And the best part? All they require is intent and herbs. We will use an extensive amount of herbs in this blend, but if you don't have them all you can substitute or choose at least five.

Rose

Lavender

Chamomile

Yarrow

Nettle

Elderflower

Passionflower

Jasmine

Lemon balm

1 mixing bowl

1 jar or container

1 clear quartz crystal

Combine all your herbs in a bowl. I recommend using your hands for this since it'll help infuse the herbs with your energy and intent.

Stir the herbs, while reciting the following chant. It doesn't matter if you stir clockwise, counterclockwise, or chaotic as fuck. I'll leave that one up to you.

"I am beautiful. I am strong. I am worthy. I am loved. I do not allow others to cloud my own self-love. I do not question myself. I am kind to my body, mind, and soul. As it was, so it shall remain."

Say it as many times as you need to. Once you feel your intent has made its point, transfer the mix from your bowl to your jar.

Place the clear quartz crystal directly in the jar, on top of the herbs, and close the lid. Store and use for up to five months.

You can use this blend:
- **As an incense:** Grab a fireproof bowl, light a small piece of charcoal, and sprinkle a pinch on top.
- **In a spell jar:** Add a lil' bit to any healing, self-love, or general mental health jars for an extra boost.
- **As a tea:** Brew 2 tablespoons (30 ml) in 8 ounces (235 ml) of water for two to three minutes.
- **As a mist or room spray base:** Brew like a tea, add a touch of rubbing alcohol, and add your chosen essential oils.
- **As a dust:** Sprinkle around your room or even around the perimeter of your home to lock in an energetic bubble of joy.

LAZY WITCH SPELLS AND RITUALS FOR
healing + self-love

A SPELL TO NOT GIVE A FUCK

LET ME TELL YOU why we're putting this spell in this chapter. Many self-love and healing issues are caused by anxiety. Anxiety is (sometimes) caused by a shitty little demon telling us that we're "not good enough to be included" or "everyone is talking shit about me" or some other bullshit. A spell to not give a fuck helps you shed that constant state of worrying over what other people think about you (or whatever the fuck your brain is making up right now). It's as easy as fuck, too, so you can do this spell pretty much whenever you want.

Any color candle

Lighter

Light your candle and whisper the following phrase into it:
"I do not give a shit. You cannot make me give a shit.
My last fuck has flown."

Blow out the candle. Use this as a symbolic way of blowing your problems away from you.

Repeat whenever you want, babe, and you can even use the same damn candle multiple times.

RESTARTING CANDLE SPELL

I KNOW EVERYONE dislikes change, but, believe me, sitting in some stagnant-ass, shitty energy is much worse. This spell will clear out all of the noise and energy you don't need or want in your general vicinity. Think of it as a mini version of a cord cutting ritual, which we'll do later in this chapter.

1 white
chime candle

Self-Love and
Healing Oil (see
page 94)

Elderflower

Clove powder

2 pieces of
paper and pen

Candle holder

Sea salt

3 pieces of
clear quartz

Lighter

Tweezers or
mini tongs

First, dress the candle with the oil (avoiding the wick). Cover your workspace with some paper towel or a plate so you don't get oil all over your surface. It's really annoying to clean up after, trust me. Rub your oil onto the candle. While rubbing, think about what we're trying to accomplish with this spell so you can low-key set some intentions as you go which, in turn, makes the spell stronger.

Mix your herbs together in a bowl, stirring it with your finger counterclockwise. Sprinkle the herbs all over the candle, making sure to stay away from the wick.

Once your candle is dressed and you've washed your hands it's time to write. This part can take anywhere from three minutes to an hour so take your time and be specific.

On one page of paper, write down everything you want gone. Any old habits, beliefs, pain, stress, emotional despair go here.

On the second page, you'll write everything you want to bring in: your hopes, dreams, emotional and spiritual goals.

Once you're done, it's time for the spell. Grab your "bring in" paper and fold it twice, away from you. This will be the first layer. Place your candle holder on top of the paper that has *everything you want to bring in* and put your dressed candle in the holder.

Make a circle around the paper and candle with your sea salt. Place the three pieces of clear quartz right outside of the circle in a triangle formation.

Light your candle and start ripping up the paper you filled out earlier with *everything you want gone.* (Rip toward you.) Grab the pieces of paper, one by one, with your teasers and burn them in the lit candle. The tweezers stop you from accidentally lighting yourself on fire and give you space to let the entire paper burn. (Pro-tip: Keep a fireproof bowl handy so you can drop the papers in if fire makes you nervous.)

As you burn the papers, repeat this chant over and over again: *"I let go of the past. I let go of everything that no longer serves me. I let go."*

Let your candle burn all the way down. Discard the ashes outside of your home, DO NOT STICK THEM IN YOUR TRASH CAN. You don't want that energy to sneak its way back.

Take the paper that was under your candle and stick it on your altar. Place a piece of clear quartz on top of it to keep the energy charged for at least twenty-four hours or up to fourteen days. Discard by burying it near the home. (Paper takes two to six weeks to decompose, but you'll forget about it before that happens, don't worry.)

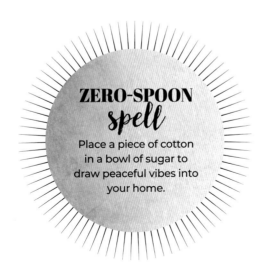

ZERO-SPOON *spell*

Place a piece of cotton in a bowl of sugar to draw peaceful vibes into your home.

CLEAN SLATE AND EMOTIONAL SUPPORT SALT BLEND

SALTS ARE SUPER versatile in witchcraft and extra easy to make. These salts are going to clear your mind and energy so you can start the day spiritually and physically clean.

You can use these salts as a bath soak or, if you absolutely hate baths, like me, because they gross you out, add the salts to a sachet and tie the sachet around your showerhead. The steam from the hot water will release all the oils and magic as you shower.

4 parts pink salt (sea salt is totally fine too)

1 part rose

1 part lavender

1 part chamomile

1 part lemon balm

2 ounces (59 ml) olive oil

20 drops of jasmine essential oil (up to 40 drops if you want the scent to be stronger)

Bowl

Gloves

6-ounce (177-ml) jar

The process is extremely straightforward. The easiest way to measure is by using your jar as the mixing bowl, to make sure it'll fit perfectly and there are no leftovers.

Start by adding the salt and herbs to your bowl. Add the salt first, then add the herbs (the order doesn't matter). While adding your salt and herbs to the jar, repeat this chant three times per ingredient: *"I live in the present. I am renewed."*

Pour the mixture into the bowl and add the oils. (If you'd like to use this as a scrub instead, add an extra 6 to 7 ounces (175-200 ml) of olive oil.)

Combine your ingredients by mixing with your hands. (Gloves are a good idea for this part or you'll smell jasmine for days.)

Store the salts in the airtight jar, and they'll have a shelf life of one to three months.

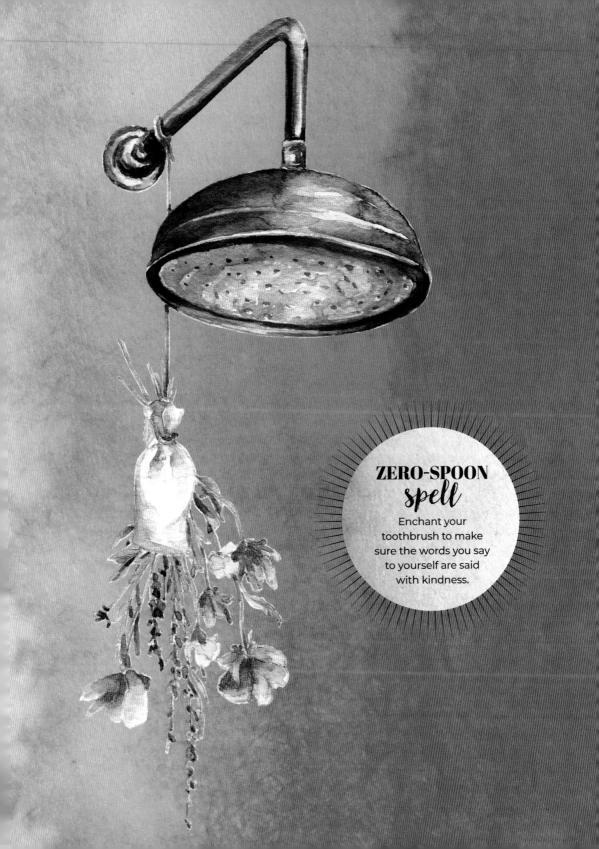

ZERO-SPOON
spell

Enchant your
toothbrush to make
sure the words you say
to yourself are said
with kindness.

CORD CUTTING FOR YOUR OLD SELF

CORD CUTTINGS ARE usually used to get rid of a connection with another person, place, or thing. This one is different, however. In this ritual, we will cut away all that shitty, trash-ass energy that your anxiety and depression hung on you, and we'll let go of past mistakes, disdain, and overall negative vibes. Because you don't have time to be up until 3 a.m. thinking about that one time in high school when you accidentally went into the boys' bathroom (I will neither confirm nor deny that this is a personal experience).

A carving tool (an old pen works)

1 white chime candle

1 black chime candle

Self-Love and Healing Oil (see page 94)

Dragon's blood incense

Sandalwood powder

2 chime candle holders

String of any kind

Fireproof plate

Start by carving your candles. On your black chime candle, carve the word "old." On the white chime candle, carve the word "new." You can take it up a notch by converting your words into sigils (see page 29) before carving them.

Next, rub a few drops of your oil into the black candle (avoiding the wick, of course) while chanting "old is past." Next, rub a few drops into your white candle while chanting "new is present."

It is time to "sprinkle, sprinkle," bitches. On your black candle, sprinkle your dragon's blood. Keep repeating "old is past" while you do this. On your white candle, sprinkle your sandalwood powder. Keep repeating "new is present" until you're done dressing.

Place each candle in its respective holder, and place the holders on your plate about 3 inches (7.5 cm) apart. Tie the string around the middle of both candles to connect the energy. It doesn't have to be tight; it just has to be tied.

Say this chant six times before lighting the candles: *"I release myself from the versions of myself I created just to survive."*

Light your candles, and watch the flames. You need to watch it the entire time for safety, so once the flame passes the string, read a book or some shit until its done because you need it to burn all the way down.

Once it's done burning, breathe. I'm dead-ass serious; here's a breathing exercise:

Breathe in through your nose for eight counts, hold for six, then breathe out through your mouth for eight. Repeat this process three times.

When you're done, discard the remnants of the spell outside of your home. You should feel lighter now. Check in with yourself in about a week to make sure the spell has worked. If you feel like you must do it again, you may. I'd wait about two to three weeks in between each session, though, kind of like when you get a facial. You don't want your face to be rubbed raw from getting one of those done every week. Don't do that to your spiritual self either. She's seen enough, okay?

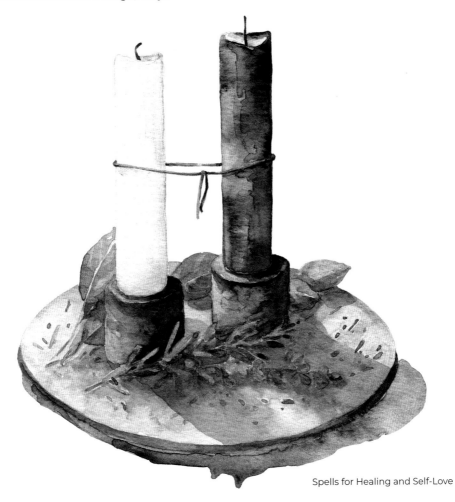

PEACEFUL AS FUCK: A DREAM SPELL

MOST DREAM SPELLS are designed to give you prophetic dreams or help your astral project. This one is specifically to help you sleep. I've had insomnia for what feels like my entire existence on this planet, and one thing that's helped me are dream spells. This spell will do a couple of things for you: help with pre-bedtime anxiety, protect you from nightmares, and assist your medications by adding magic to make them more potent.

Pink salt

Rose

Passionflower

Elderflower

Clear, glass bowl

Moon water (see page 19)

3 pieces of tumbled moonstone

Take yourself and your ingredients over to your nightstand because that's where we'll be making the entire spell. If you don't have a nightstand, sit your happy ass right on the floor next to your bed. (Just make sure it's not where you step when you wake up in the morning because no one likes wet feet.)

There is one chant you'll repeat for the entirety of this spell: *"I am safe. I am calm. I am peace. I am rest."*

Repeat this at least one time for each step.

Add your herbs to the bowl one by one, stirring them counterclockwise to combine. Next, pour enough moon water into the bowl to make the herbs float (you should not need to fill it all the way). Place the moonstones around the bowl in a triangle formation.

Stir everything clockwise, eight times. I know, it's specific, but eight hours is the "normal" recommended amount of sleep time. Eight stirs, eight hours.

And that's it! Turn off the lights and go to sleep.

You can reuse the same bowl for about three nights before it starts to mold. If you'd like to keep it fresh for a couple more days, add in a splash of rubbing alcohol.

Discard the contents outside of your home. It basically captured all the energy you didn't want near you.

STRESS BREAKER, SEA SHAKER JAR

WHETHER YOUR STRESS comes from financial strain, health issues, family problems, or literally anything else life throws at us, this jar will lend a helping hand and ground you in the moment. It's inspired by the sea. The sea is calming and soothing and brings you back to the moment, keeping you grounded as fuck. If you don't happen to live by the ocean, switch your sea water with moon water.

Sandalwood

Skullcap

Lemon balm

Nettle

Lavender

Chamomile

Any blue crystal chips (blue lace agate is recommended but not required)

Sea shells (optional)

Sea water or moon water

Rubbing alcohol

A jar with a lid

Lighter

1 blue candle

Start by adding your herbs in following order: sandalwood, skullcap, lemon balm, nettle, lavender, chamomile. While you add them, repeat this chant once per herb: *"Endless sea, allow me to only see joy and positivity."*

Add your crystal chips. If you've opted to use seashells, you'll add those in now as well.

Add in your water and rubbing alcohol. Use a 10:1 ratio to prevent molding. As your pour the water in, say: *"Like water flows, so does my happiness."*

Place the lid on your jar. Light your candle and seal it by dripping the wax around the lid. Be sure to cover every crevice as this will add an extra layer of protection, metaphorically and literally. You don't want the water or energy spilling out at any point.

And you're done! Keep the jar on your altar, in your office, on your nightstand, in the kitchen, basically wherever the fuck you want.

Shake it when you're stressed the fuck out to activate the magic. Remake every three months.

A SPELL FOR SAD DAYS

EVEN IF YOU don't normally suffer from depression, we all have our days. You know, the days where you feel like you're being crushed under the weight of existing in this dystopian hellscape? (Okay, I'm being dramatic, but you get my point.) This spell is for those days.

 This spell is meant to be done OUTDOORS. I know, it's scary out there. I often get a bit of anxiety when there's a possibility that someone might see me doing weird witchcraft shit, so it's totally fine, I get it. Just go on your porch if you're feeling anxious about that part.

1 carving tool

1 orange, gold, or yellow candle

Lighter

1 plate (heat-resistant, please and thank you)

3 small, raw citrine chunks

3 small tumbled sunstone pieces

Lemon balm

Chamomile

Calendula

Passionflower

1 small sachet (any color except black)

First, gather your shit and go the fuck outside. Do some breathing exercises to calm any anxieties you might have. This spell will be done completely on the floor, so you don't even need a chair. (But if a chair is required, that's totally fine.)

Once you're nice and calm, carve the sun symbol onto your candle. The sun symbol is literally just a circle with a dot in the middle. Nothing crazy, don't overthink it.

Melt the bottom of your candle slightly and stick it to the middle of your plate. Place your crystals around the perimeter. If your plate is big enough, place them directly on it. If not, place them on the ground around it.

Sprinkle your herbs on the plate, keeping them inside the circle you made with your crystals.

Light your candle and start chanting, babe. Say each line three times.

"I can overcome anything. I have made it through
*   100 percent of my bad days, and I can do it again.*
I am gentle with myself. I am doing the best I can in the
*   situations I have been given.*
I believe in a better tomorrow. I can change my life,
*   one step at a time.*
My thoughts do not define me. I am confident
*   and remember that our minds play tricks.*
I am enough. I was enough. I will always be enough and
*   that is enough."*

When the candle has burnt out and cooled down, scoop up all your ingredients (including the leftover candle wax, if there is any) and place everything into your sachet.

Keep the sachet on your altar for three days. Repeat this spell whenever your depression monster decides it's time to play again.

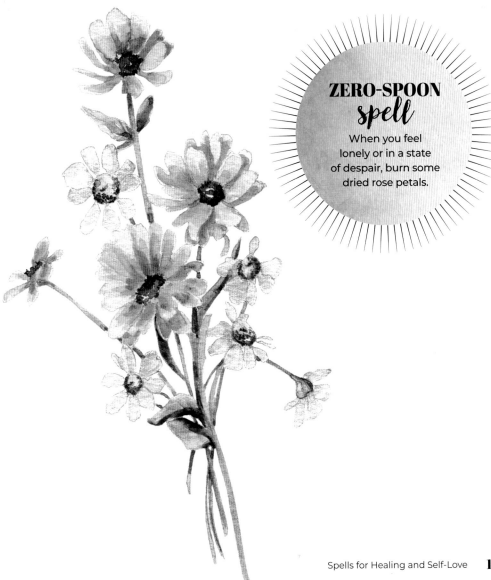

ZERO-SPOON
spell

When you feel lonely or in a state of despair, burn some dried rose petals.

APHRODITE'S GLAMOUR TEA

THIS ISN'T YOUR normal "make me pretty" glamour. This is a glamour for those of us who enjoy socializing but get too anxious or self-conscious about every little thing that happens. Think of this tea as a veil. Usually, you wear a veil to stop others from taking or adding to your energy, but this veil will act like an anxiety blanket. It will help you socialize easier by assisting your brain in not thinking that the world is ending because you accidentally broke a glass or someone looked at you weirdly.

6 ounces (175 ml) water

1 tablespoon (15 g) chamomile

1 tablespoon (15 g) lemon balm

1 teaspoon (5 g) lavender

1 teaspoon (5 g) jasmine

1 teaspoon (5 g) hibiscus

Tea strainer

Tea cup

Honey and lemon, to taste

While the water boils, combine all the herbs in a strainer. (Yeah, I know, most of us will just stick that shit in the microwave, but let's just pretend we're all functioning members of society.)

As the water boils, hold the strainer filled with the tea mix in your hands and recite this chant four times: *"Aphrodite, goddess of love, give me the same faith you have in me. Give me the gift of controlling what I can and letting go of what I can't. Protect me from the thoughts of others and only allow truth inside my aura. So it is said, so it shall be."*

Stick your strainer in your teacup and pour in the boiled water.

Let it steep for two to four minutes. Add honey and lemon as needed or desired, but remember to stir clockwise for this one.

Drink like normal and be free of other people's negative thinking, my children.

BREAK-UP SHOWER RITUAL

ONE OF THE most powerful ways to cleanse your energy is by visualizing while you shower. When we combine that with herbs, crystals, and tools, the results are truly noticeable. And who the fuck doesn't want to be cleansed of their shitty ex's energy? Who would want to keep that? Like, have you met our exes? Be for real. Anyway, this ritual will take good care of you, babe.

1 sachet

Sea salt

Passionflower

Lavender

Rose

30 drops of sandalwood essential oil

Rose quartz chunk

A shower

Start by making your shower sachet. Add in each ingredient to the sachet one a time while saying the following phrases:

"Sea salt helps me start fresh and new
Passionflower will calm and soothe me.
Lavender will cleanse and purify me.
Rose will fill the room with love.
Sandalwood will help deal with, support, and
*   understand my emotions.*
Rose quartz will amplify all of the herbal energies."

You can add a few more drops of your sandalwood oil to the outside of the pouch for some more aromatherapy.

Head on over to your shower and set a mood. You can play soothing music, light a candle or two, add some crystals, etc.

Tie the sachet around your showerhead and start your shower.

This next part is meant to be done AFTER you've finished all your usual showering necessities, like shampooing your hair and washing behind your ears. Take a minute and look directly at the water coming out of the showerhead. (Don't let it hit your eyes, though, because that would be bad for your ocular health.) Imagine a white light replacing the water droplets. Imagine the white light showering you in warmth and happiness.

Look down at the drain, and imagine the water that's going down it is gray and generally unappealing. Switch from looking at the drain to the showerhead and vice versa for one to three minutes.

Almost in exact synchrony with the motion of turning the handle to end your shower, say: *"I am cleansed."*

Discard the sachet outside of your home.

THE EASIEST EMOTIONAL HEALING CHARM

LITERALLY, THIS SPELL is the easiest one I could come up with. When we're emotional, we rarely have any concern or desire to do anything. This is the closest thing I can give you to nothing.

Self-Love and Healing Oil (see page 94)

2 pink candles

1 rose quartz chunk

Rub a few drops of the Self-Love and Healing Oil onto your candles (avoiding the wicks, of course). Set the candles directly on your work surface or in candle holders about 5 inches (13 cm) apart. Place your rose quartz in the middle of the two candles.

Light your candles, and let the rose quartz absorb the healing and loving energy coming from the candles.

Once the candles are done burning, hold your crystal in your hands. Say: *"I am not my past. I am not my mistakes. I am not stupid. I am not alone. I am worthy."*

Keep your crystal with you at all times (or as much as you can).

Recharge by repeating the same ritual every one to two weeks.

RISE AND SHINE, BITCHES: A SPELL FOR THE MORNING

MORNINGS ARE LITERALLY the fucking worst. For this spell, we'll basically make ourselves a little spiritual wake-up call that'll help us start the day off with a bit more happiness and joy. This spell is meant to be made the day before (afternoonish), because, honestly, nobody wakes up and says, "Ya know what? A magical ritual at the ass-crack of dawn sounds like a great idea."

Citrine

Sunstone

Rose quartz

Bowl

Sea salt

Sun water

Yarrow

Jasmine

1 pouch (yellow preferred, but any color is fine)

Place your crystals in your bowl one by one while chanting their respective intentions:

*"Citrine, bring me happiness,
Sunstone, bring me joy.
Rose quartz, bring me unconditional love for myself."*

Pour the sea salt on top of the crystals. It doesn't need to cover them completely, just enough to fill the bottom of the bowl. Say: *"With this salt, I amplify my intent."*

Pour three drops of sunwater onto each crystal. Say: *"Apollo, bring me the warmth of the sun."*

Next, sprinkle the yarrow and jasmine into the bowl. Say: *"Yarrow, bring me bliss. Jasmine, bring everything in this bowl into pure harmony and balance, so mote it be."*

Leave the bowl in the sunlight as it sets. As soon as you see the sun disappear, bring it back inside. (Use a weather app or website to see when the sun goes down in your area. Set an alarm or reminder to bring it out and another to bring it in. Trust me.)

Once you're back inside, pour the contents from your bowl into your pouch. Hang the pouch ABOVE your bedroom door frame (on the outer side). You can use push pins so you don't have giant nail holes on your wall. The pouch will infuse your aura with the energy and intent you placed on it when you walk out of your bedroom in the morning.

You can reuse this spell for three weeks before needing to refresh or redo the pouch.

SIMMER UP JOY

SIMMER POTS ARE one of my easiest hacks when you want potent magic but don't want to set anything on fire or keep an eye on it. You can customize them to fit multiple intentions; this one will be for happiness, love, peace, and joy.

People always ask me if you can ingest the liquid after it's finished. While you are welcome to try this, you will need to figure out measurements for the ingredients that will actually taste good, as this recipe is not specific enough to be consumed as is.

Decent-size pot

4 bay leaves

Wooden spoon

Moon water

Orange slices

Cinnamon sticks

Roses

Lemon slices

Lavender

Apple pie spice (optional, for fragrance)

Place your pot on the stove and add in your water until it's around 60 percent full. Turn the heat on medium, and let it come to a boil while we do the next step.

Make either a sigil for the following intention (see page 29) or just write the intention word directly on the bay leaves. (I would opt for sigils if you don't live alone.) The intentions are "peace," "joy," "happiness," and "love." Use one bay leaf for each one.

Once your water starts to boil, turn the heat down to keep the water at a simmer. It's a fucking simmer pot, not a "let's boil the tears of my enemies" pot.

Adding the ingredients one by one, and repeat the four intentions in your head (or out loud, but I'm not responsible for your roommates' stares) as you do so. Remember, the measurements are fully up to you. Leave the bay leaves until last.

Once all the other ingredients have been added to the pot, crush your bay leaves in your hands, one by one, before throwing them in your pot.

And that is all the work you have to do until you're ready to discard the water.

You can leave this on super low heat for four to five hours. DON'T EVER LEAVE YOUR STOVE ON WHEN YOU'RE NOT HOME.

When you are ready to discard the simmer pot, you can do one of two things. First, you can simply toss it outside of your home because it's essentially collected all the energy you didn't want left in your home. Or second, you can strain the herbs and

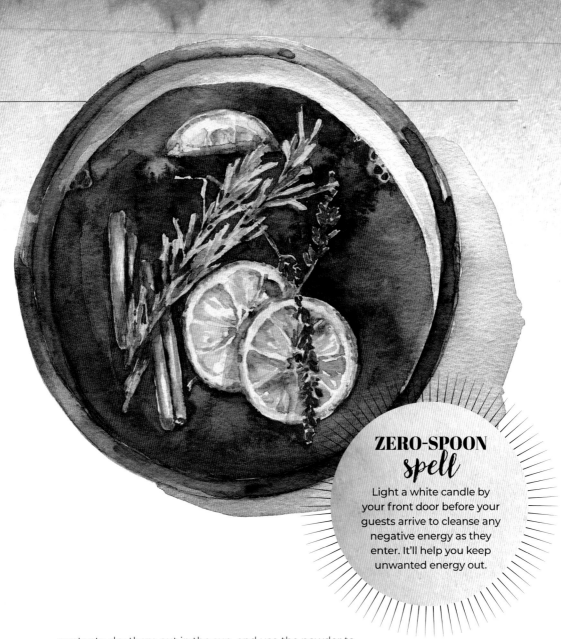

ZERO-SPOON
spell
Light a white candle by your front door before your guests arrive to cleanse any negative energy as they enter. It'll help you keep unwanted energy out.

contents, dry them out in the sun, and use the powder to make a "happy, joyful" salt blend. Kind of like black salt, but less aggressive.

I do this spell once a month if I am feeling up to it, but once a year totally works too. (Do not tell my mom, though—she thinks I do it every other week.)

AURA CLEANSING SUGAR SCRUB

OUR AURAS ARE super sensitive and the people, places, and things we surround ourselves with all have the potential to cause holes, rips, or stagnant energy. This scrub will cleanse the negative bullshit, get rid of heavy unwanted energy, and let your real aura come to light.

Mixing bowl

½ cup (118 ml) regular household sugar

Clear quartz

Rose

Elderflower

Chamomile

Yarrow

4 ounces (120 ml) fractionated coconut oil (see note)

30 drops of jasmine essential oil (see note)

6-ounce (168 g) container

Grab your bowl and measure out your sugar. Stick your clear quartz crystal in the middle of the bowl of sugar. Let it sit there for a couple minutes while repeating this chant to allow the quartz to charge the sugar with your intent: *"Aura cleanse, aura new. Aura filled with light and all things good."*

Add the herbs one by one, envisioning a white light radiating off of them as you sprinkle them in. You can repeat the following phrase if visualization isn't your strong suit or if you just don't have the mental strength for all that right now: *"Get this shitty energy all the way the fuck out. Cleanse my aura and clear my self-doubts."*

Once your herbs are in, give it a quick mix, then add your coconut oil. If you have sensitive skin, you can add jojoba or vitamin E oils to help your skin and your aura at the same time.

Thoroughly mix the coconut oil in the blend, then add your jasmine essential oil and mix some more, babe.

Remove the quartz from the bowl and pour the contents of the bowl into your jar. If you have enough space left in the jar, you can actually keep the crystal in there for up to seven days. The shelf life for this scrub is between two to four weeks. When you're finished, you can make it again or reuse the jar for another spell.

Note: If you've got sensitive skin and don't want to use essential oil, switch it out with its herbal counterpart.

DIVINE RADIANCE LEMONADE

THIS TEA-TURNED-LEMONADE will boost your confidence, raise your vibrations, and make you radiate divine energy.

2 tablespoons (28 g) rosehip

2 tablespoons (28 g) rose petals

1 teaspoon (5 g) hibiscus

1 teaspoon (5 g) elderflower

Mixing bowl

5 cups (1.175 ml) water, divided

1 cup (235 ml) sugar

Strainer or cheesecloth

1¾ cup (410 ml) lemon juice

Lemon

16-ounce (454-g) pitcher

First, combine your herbs in a bowl. Once they're combined, wave your hand over the bowl three times while chanting: *"Divine Goddesses, lend me some of your radiance. Let me see myself in a brighter light, the way you see me. As it is said, so it shall be. I thank thee."*

Pour 3 cups (710 ml) of water into a pot and bring to a boil. Pour the herb mix directly into the pot and turn the stove off. Let the herbs steep for ten to fifteen minutes.

Add your sugar while the herbs are steeping and mix until you see no sugar left.

Once the tea is fully steeped, strain out the herbs completely. You won't be happy if you accidentally eat a piece of elderflower or something. Let the tea cool completely before moving on.

When the tea is cool, add the lemon juice and the rest of the water. Then transfer it to your pitcher. Place your pitcher in the fridge and let it chill.

Drink as normal. As you sip, feel the divine energy entering your body. This lemonade has a shelf life of three to five days.

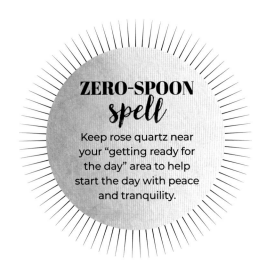

ZERO-SPOON *spell*

Keep rose quartz near your "getting ready for the day" area to help start the day with peace and tranquility.

SELF-LOVE ROSARY

ROSARIES HAVE BEEN used for centuries for spirituality and religious purposes. You're familiar with the Catholic rosary, right? Think that, but make it witchy. I did not specify a type of bead for this spell because we're all on different budgets. However, I do have a few suggestions. Remember this is your own version so you can choose any beads and any pattern you'd like. Rose quartz and blue lace agate beads would be ideal with a few wooden beads thrown in. If you can't get the gemstone beads, stick to wood or lava rock. You can add a few drops of essential oil to the wood and lava beads to make it an aromatherapy experience.

20 to 30 beads

Small plate

Self-Love Herb Blend (see page 96)

String

Before you start going wild stringing beads all willy nilly, let's charge them, yeah? Pour some of the Self-Love Herb Blend directly onto a plate. Place the beads on top of the herbs and let them charge for 2 to 3 hours. Separate your herbs from your beads when you feel the energy is right. Keep the plate of herbs to the side. Now you're ready to begin assembling.

Start stringing your charged beads onto the string one by one. As you add each bead, imagine them radiating a white light that gets brighter every time you add a new one. Once you've added all your beads, close the necklace by tying both ends together but leave a small space so you can move the beads around as you go through your affirmations.

Extra credit: You can add a small charm to the string to give you the same starting point each time you use them.

Now let's go over how to use your Self-Love Rosary. You'll recite affirmations for each bead. You can choose one affirmation and repeat it or mix it up, or do a different one for each bead—that part is up to you. I've included ten affirmations to get you started; however, the more you create and use your own affirmations, the more intention will go into the prayer.

Start by holding the beads in your hands for a few minutes, while you do a breathing exercise or mini meditation just to get in the mood. When you're ready, start reciting your affirmations, holding one of the beads at a time, and switching to the next bead in the line when you're done with the last one. That's it.

Sample Affirmations for Self-Love:
- I am the god of my reality, and I create all the beautiful things I deserve.
- I am worthy of love.
- I choose myself before other people I care about.
- I am proud of everything I've accomplished despite the fire I had to walk through to get here.
- I am beautiful and radiate confidence.
- I am unique; there is only one of me on this planet.
- I am my own hero; everything I need comes from within.
- I apologize to my body when I am hard on it.
- I appreciate everything my body, mind, and soul has gotten me through.
- I am enough just the way I am.

Store on top of the same small plate with the herb mix and leave it on your altar. Use it whenever you need a self-loving boost.

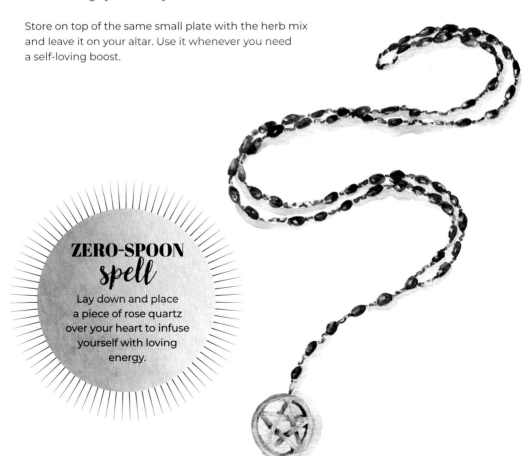

ZERO-SPOON
spell
Lay down and place a piece of rose quartz over your heart to infuse yourself with loving energy.

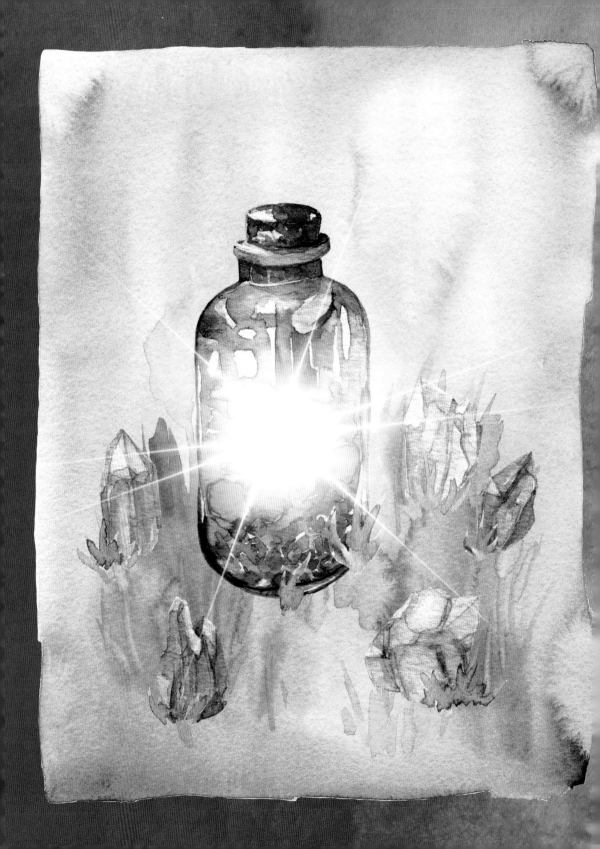

5

SPELLS FOR
focus + energy

There have been years of my life where 90 percent of my spells were for focus and energy. If you're reading this book, I'm just going to go ahead and assume you're like me and you're constantly tired. If your energy is low, it affects your relationships, your work, your creativity, your spirituality, and your witchcraft.

Imagine your energy as a light. That light is what powers your witchcraft. When you're unfocused and tired, your light dims, which in turn makes your spells and rituals less effective. Doing energy, focus, or creativity spells replenishes that light.

MATERIALS AND CORRESPONDENCES FOR LAZY WITCH
focus, energy, creativity + the sun

CORRESPONDENCES FOR SOLAR ENERGY, ENERGY, FOCUS, AND CREATIVITY

	Solar Energy	General Energy
Moon Phase	Bitch, there's no moon correspondence here. It's literally the sun.	Full
Zodiac	Aries, Cancer, Leo	Aries, Leo, Sagittarius, Scorpio
Colors	Gold, yellow, purple, white, orange, brown	Blue, brown, copper, grey, green, orange, red, yellow
Day of the Week	Sunday	Tuesday
Tarot Card	Strength, Sun	Emperor, Strength
Herbs, Plants, and Flowers	Birch, cedar, hazelnut, juniper, marigold, rosemary, St. John's wort, sunflower, olive leaf, angelica, chamomile, chrysanthemum, clove, frankincense, galangal	Elderflower, elderberry, juniper, oak, pine, agrimony, basil, catnip, chamomile, fill, fennel, marigold, peppermint, rose, St. John's wort, sunflower, thyme, all spice, burdock root, clove, frankincense, galangal, orris root, ginger, nettle, nutmeg, vanilla
Crystals and Gemstones	Amber, calcite, carnelian, citrine, peridot, quartz, sunstone, tiger's eye, black tourmaline	Amber, aventurine, orange calcite, carnelian, citrine, garnet, hematite, red jasper, yellow jasper, kyanite, selenite, smoky quartz, pyrite, sunstone, tiger's eye

In this chapter, our intentions revolve around energy, creativity, and focus. We'll work with the sun a lot here to help you feel energized and ready to tackle any task you have ahead of you—even when you really don't feel like doing shit (or you do, but your brain just won't let you).

Below, you'll find a correspondence table for each intention. Don't worry—you won't need every item in this chart for the spells and rituals in the chapter. This is a master list of EVERYTHING so that you have plenty of alternatives in case you don't have a specific correspondence for a spell or ritual you want to perform.

You can see that our correspondence table has a good amount of overlap between the various intentions. To narrow things down further, the following tables list all the ingredients you'll need for the spells in this chapter, along with their substitutions (to save you time, money, and extra effort if you're missing anything). As a rule, you can switch out the essential oils for their solid counterparts.

Focus	Creativity
Full	Full, waning, waxing
Capricorn	Aquarius, Gemini, Leo, Pisces, Scorpio
Brown, red, violet, white, yellow	Black, gold, green, orange, pink, red, white, yellow
Tuesday	Monday, Sunday, Wednesday
Chariot	Empress, Magician
Cardamom, cinnamon, frankincense, myrrh, sutmeg, sandalwood, skullcap, vanilla, bas, bergamot, garlic, hibiscus, lavender, lemon balm, peppermint, rosemary, spearmint	Birch bark, cherry bark, elderberries, hawthorn leaf, pine, pomegranate, chamomile, jasmine, lavender, peppermint, rose, rosemary, vervain, cardamom, cinnamon, clove, lotus, mushroom, nutmeg, orris root, patchouli, sandalwood, skullcap
Amazonite, amethyst, bloodstone, calcite, carnelian, fluorite, hematite, kyanite, lepidolite, snowflake obsidian, pyrite, clear quartz	Agate, amber, aquamarine, aventurine, orange calcite, chrysocolla, citrine, emerald, fluorite, garnet, howlite, jasper, lapis lazuli, moonstone, moss agate, obsidian, opalite, tiger's eye

PLANTS, HERBS, AND FLOWERS

Ingredient	Substitution
Basil	Nettle
Bay leaves	Allspice
Calendula	Sunflower
Chrysanthemum	Chamomile
Cinnamon	Nutmeg
Frankincense	Copal
Ginger	Galangal root
Lemongrass	Lemon peel
Orris root	Patchouli
Peppermint	Eucalyptus
Frankincense	Myrrh
Rosemary	Thyme
Willow bark	Olive leaf

CARRIER OILS AND ESSENTIAL OILS

Ingredient	Substitution
Cedarwood essential oil	Juniper essential oil
Clove essential oil	Cinnamon essential oil
Olive oil	Sunflower or coconut oil

CRYSTALS AND GEMSTONES

Ingredient	Substitution
Carnelian (chips and chunks)	Orange calcite
Citrine (chips and chunks)	Fluorite
Red jasper (chunks)	Yellow jasper
Sunstone (chips)	Mookaite
Tiger's eye (chips)	Lapis lazuli

OTHER SHIT

Ingredient	Substitution
Cinnamon sticks	Clove or anise
Coffee grounds	Green tea
Frankincense	Myrrh
Sea salt	Table salt

BASIC TEALIGHTS, SIGILS, AND OIL BLENDS
focus + energy

By now you know the drill. The following tealights, sigils, and oil blends are simple and adaptable—the perfect standbys for really shitty days when one or two spoons is literally all you have to give.

The two oils in this section will be the base for a few spells throughout the chapter. But you don't have to save them just for spellwork. You can rub that shit all over yourself, your tools, or whatever else whenever you feel like you need boost. For an extra wild ride, combine both oils when anointing your body or tools.

TWO-INGREDIENT TEALIGHTS FOR FOCUS AND ENERGY

Tealight

Herbs and Crystals:

- Focus: peppermint and citrine chips
- Creativity: orange peel and carnelian chips
- Energy: rosemary and peppermint

Set your intentions for what you want the spell to bring you. Light the tealight and let the wax melt a bit. Blow it out when you have a melty surface. Sprinkle your herbs and chips on top of the melted wax, being very careful and cautious to not let the herb near the flame. Save your tealight for later or light it right away.

SIGILS FOR FOCUS AND ENERGY

CREATE A SIGIL based on your intentions for focus and energy and use them as follows. (As a reminder, for full instructions on how to make a sigil, see Chapter 1, page 29.)

- Draw "ENERGY" on the bottom of your shoes.
- Draw "CREATIVITY" on your pencil case or holder.
- Draw "FOCUS" on your laptop case or notebook.

FIRE AND FOCUS OIL

STIMULATE YOUR CREATIVITY and let those inventive thoughts and feelings manifest into energy.

Paper and pen

⅓-ounce (10-ml) empty dropper or rollerball

Sunstone chips

Rosemary

Cinnamon sticks

20 drops of clove essential oil

Sunflower oil

On a piece of paper, write: *"With fire by my side, my focus will not subside."*

Place the paper on your altar with all of your raw ingredients on top. Let the paper charge your ingredients for thirty minutes to ten hours. It totally depends on you and how you feel at the moment of charging. You can even do it the day before.

Grab your dropper or rollerball and add your ingredients. Start with your chips, then herbs, then sticks, then essential oil, and finish with the sunflower oil, which you'll fill to the top. Close the top securely and shake eleven times. As you shake, repeat the chant you wrote earlier eleven times.

Use the oil on your pressure points whenever you feel tired, out of it, or just want to give your brain a lil' boost.

ANTI-PROCRASTINATION OIL

STOP SAYING, "OH I CAN DO THAT LATER," because we both know you won't, in fact, be doing that later.

Small mason jar

Basil

Peppermint

Rosemary

10 drops of lemon essential oil

15 drops of orange essential oil

Sunflower oil

10-ml (⅓-ounce) empty rollerball

Add your ingredients to a mason jar starting with the herbs, then the essential oils, then the sunflower oil. Set your intentions by telling them what they're doing while putting them in the jar:

"Basil, you will to ground me in the moment.
Peppermint and rosemary, you will awaken my inner bad bitch.
Lemon and orange, you will cleanse all the random thoughts
* flying around in my head.*
Sunflower oil, you will bind everyone together to create the
* perfect blend."*

Once everything has been added, screw the lid of the jar on tight and shake chaotically to get the energy flowing.

Leave your jar in a cool, dark place for at least three days (a full week is better). Once it's infused, fill your rollerball from the jar and use normally. You can strain the herbs if you'd like, but it's not a requirement.

This oil doesn't really go bad so you can keep the rest of the oil in its jar in a cool, dark place and refill your rollerball as needed.

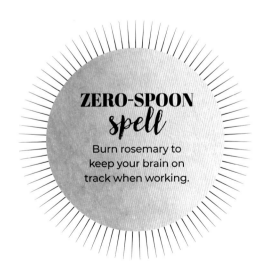

ZERO-SPOON
spell

Burn rosemary to keep your brain on track when working.

LAZY WITCH SPELLS AND RITUALS FOR
focus + energy

CLARITY SHAKER JAR

SOMETIMES OUR MINDS get so full of the random information we take in all day that it's hard to figure out which thoughts come from us, which thoughts come from our mood, which come from our guides, and which come from outside influences. This jar will give you a way to settle all the thoughts and bring you that little bit of clarity you need to get through the task at hand.

1 empty jar with lid

Peppermint

Rosemary

Orris root

Ginger root

Tiger's eye chips

Sun water

Rubbing alcohol

Biodegradable glitter (optional)

1 yellow candle

Cleanse your chosen jar with smoke or sound. Add in your ingredients, starting with the herbs and ending with the chips. As you stick them in the jar, tell each item what the fuck it's doing here.

"Peppermint, clear my mind from all the clutter.
Rosemary, help me focus on what needs to be done.
Orris root, keep me on the right track to accomplish these tasks.
Ginger root, energize my mind and keep me alert.
Tiger's eye, give me the confidence I need to keep any in myself
  doubts at bay."

Fill your jar about three-quarters with the sun water and the rest with rubbing alcohol; the alcohol stops the water from molding because moldy energy is not what we need.

For a bonus, add biodegradable glitter to the jar give it a snow globe effect. It doesn't add much magic, but it does add happiness, which is technically magic.

Stick your lid back on. Light the yellow candle and pour a little wax onto the lid of the jar to seal it. If the candle is not yellow, that's cool. White works also.

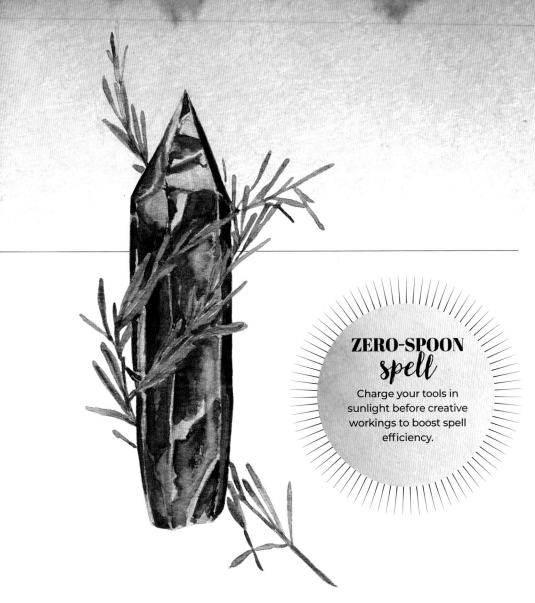

ZERO-SPOON
spell

Charge your tools in
sunlight before creative
workings to boost spell
efficiency.

Whenever you feel foggy or have executive dysfunction (don't
worry, I'm not judging you), shake the jar to activate the energy
and watch everything inside settle. Once it's settled, you should
be ready to tackle the task.

Note: You'll have to recharge the jar in the sunlight for a few hours
once a week, but just stick it in your window. You don't even need
to leave your house.

MOTIVATION CANDLE SPELL

HAVE YOU EVER had energy out the ass but absolutely no will to do anything? Gotta clean your house, but just don't want to? Need to change a light bulb, but honestly it seems like a lot? This spell is for when you're ready to say "fuck you" to all of that. Let's get some shit done.

1 orange or yellow candle

Anti-Procrastination Oil (see page 125)

Olive oil

Coffee grounds

Orange peel, grated

Candle holder

3 pieces of citrine

First, grab a plate or a paper towel to place underneath your candle so you don't have to clean up random oil spots later. (Pro tip: Rubbing alcohol cleans up oil easily.)

Put your candle on your work surface and rub your anti-procrastination oil onto it (avoiding the wick, of course).

Sprinkle your coffee grounds on the candle and say loudly, *"Wake me the fuck up!"* Try not to draw attention; we don't want you to end up in the loony bin, babe.

Sprinkle your orange peel next and say, *"Keep me fucking focused, bitch."*

Place the candle in the candle holder, then arrange the citrine around it in a triangle formation with the candle in the middle. As you light it, say, *"Drive away the fucking delays."*

You can let it burn all the way down now or blow it out when you're ready and relight it the next time you feel the need for some extra motivation.

INTELLIGENCE ENHANCING SACHET

SOMETIMES YOU WANT to learn everything at once. (When you're neurospicy, it's even worse because it can become such a long list that it's honestly discouraging.) This sachet will help keep from you getting discouraged when you're feeling distracted by ALL THE THINGS and remind you to stay on track and take it one step at a time.

Paper and pen

Any pouch
or sachet
(you can use a
random piece of
fabric, too)

1 bay leaf

Peppermint

Rosemary

Willow bark

Cedarwood oil

Lavender, orange,
or yellow string

First, grab your pen and paper; it's time to write some shit. Write everything you want to learn. Everything. It doesn't matter if it's now, later, never, or maybe. Write it the fuck down. Take your time; make it as short or long as you want.

Fold the paper three times toward you to bring that energy in. Add it to your pouch or sachet.

Add your bay leaf next. Say: *"With this leaf, wishes come true."*

Add your peppermint. Say: *"With this mint, I am focused on my goals."*

Add your rosemary. Say: *"With this herb, my guides will keep me on the right track."*

Add your willow bark. Say: *"With this bark, knowledge flows to me easily."*

Finally, add a few drops of cedarwood oil and say: *"And just in case, here's some luck."*

Tie your string around your sachet at least three times. Keep it on your desk or in your backpack.

ZERO-SPOON *spell*

Tie a yellow string around your laptop cord for heightened concentration.

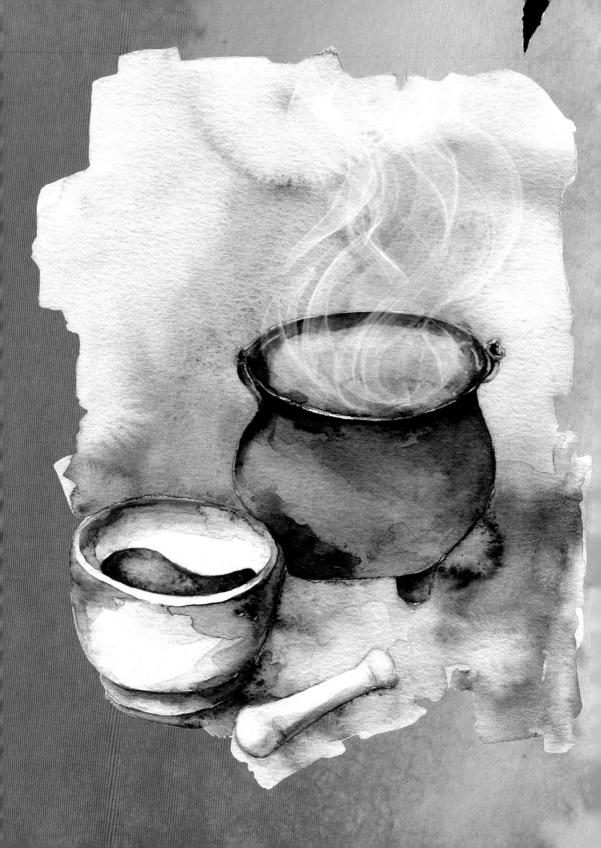

ENERGIZING CAULDRON SPELL

WHETHER YOU'RE TIRED because you haven't slept or because you work too much, energy is needed to survive in this bitch-ass world. Coffee is cool, but your spirit might not respond to your forty-fifth cup this week, so maybe try this energizing cauldron spell instead.

Paper and pen

1 piece of charcoal

Tongs or tweezers

A cauldron or fireproof bowl

Ginger

Cinnamon

Small jar

First, write down all the shit you need to get done today or during the whole week. It's up to you how much you want to write and how long you want the spell to last. You don't need to fill a whole paper, but you can if you want. It's your spell, bitch; you do you.

Once you're done, cut or rip your sheet into small pieces. The pieces will be burned in the bowl so make them small enough to fit. You don't want the paper to catch fire and accidentally fall out of the bowl. That's how we get forest fires (or home fires) and only you can prevent them.

Grab the charcoal with tongs or tweezers, light it, and place it in the cauldron. Add your paper pieces one by one. You don't need to wait for each one to burn fully before adding the next one—just fucking do it.

Next, grab a pinch of each herb and sprinkle it on there, repeating this affirmation: *"Energy flows through me as easily as it travels through the universe. My energy is restored with each positive move I make. I have the energy to complete these tasks."*

Let the charcoal burn all the way out and allow it to cool fully before moving on. Be patient, bitch, or you'll burn yourself on the next step.

When the charcoal is fully burnt out and cooled, collect the ash in your jar and sprinkle it around you or your general vicinity (desk, car, floor) when you need a boost while completing your work. (I just sprinkle it whenever I'm starting a new task, but it's totally up to you.)

SPARK ENERGY AMULET

WHEN YOU DON'T have energy to do a spell for energy, this is a great way to have something in your hands, ready to go at a moment's notice. The amulet only needs to be recharged once every fifth use, making it even more perfect.

Peppermint

Rosemary

Coffee grounds

Sea salt

Any bowl (if its gold or yellow, that would be perfect)

Any necklace or keychain you love to use

Add the herbs to the bowl one at a time. Before you add each one, hold it in your hand and whisper the following affirmation to infuse the energy you want: *"Energy flows through and around me, like waves crashing on the shore. Focus anchors me like the moon directing the tides."*

Once everything is in your bowl, stir the mix clockwise to bring the energy in. Place your necklace or keychain in the bowl, directly in the middle. Take your bowl outside on a sunny day and let it charge for three to five hours.

Once it's charged, your amulet is ready to use. Wear it or keep it with you whenever you're going to a place that requires energy. You can save the leftover herbs in a jar so you can recharge the amulet every one to two weeks.

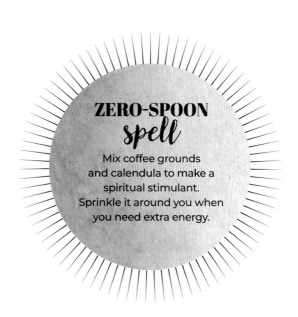

ZERO-SPOON *spell*

Mix coffee grounds and calendula to make a spiritual stimulant. Sprinkle it around you when you need extra energy.

RESET THAT SHIT ROOM MIST

SOMETIMES ENERGY GETS STUCK, which can make us feel so overwhelmed that we have absolutely no direction in our life, our work, our art. It's an easy fix, though. Just use this spray in any room that needs to be reset. You can also use it in your car or office or in public (people might look at you funny, but WHO CARES?).

Moon water

Rubbing alcohol (or polysorbate or vodka)

Citrine chips

Calendula flowers

Rosemary

Basil

Peppermint

Grated orange peel

Your favorite essential oil or fragrance oil

Spray bottle (amber is preferred, any color accepted)

Small jar with lid

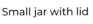

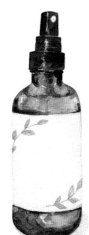

This will take about two days to make, so mentally prepare yourself for that shit (I know, I'm sorry, but you will spend most of it waiting for the spell to charge, so the work itself isn't too bad.)

Day one is easy. Add all of your herbs in your jar. Tell each herb why it's here to set your intentions as you add them to the jar:

"Calendula flowers, you're the main resetting ingredient. Rosemary, you're going to cleanse the fuck out of this energy. Basil, you're going to give us some fresh and new beginnings. Peppermint, you're going to give us clarity to see what we need to let go of. Orange peel, you'll be blessing this entire mix."

Fill the jar with rubbing alcohol and moon water at a 1-to-3 ratio.

Place the jar in the moonlight to charge overnight. BE PATIENT. Waiting is the hardest part.

The next day, add your citrine chips to your spray bottle. Tell them why they're there.

"Citrine, you'll bring me balance, harmony, and healing."

Strain the herbs from your mixture, then pour the liquid into your bottle. Repeat the following affirmation while adding the liquid: *"With this mix, I invite positivity to my life. With this mix, I invite energy into my life. With this mix, my space will feel like my space again."*

Complete the spell by adding a few drops of your favorite essential oil or fragrance and spray away, babe.

This spray will last two to three weeks at room temperature or two to four weeks in the fridge.

LIGHT SUMMONING JAR

CREATIVITY REQUIRES A good amount of energy to achieve a final result. This is where my light summoning jar comes in. We're basically summoning as much light energy as we can into a jar. You can keep it in your art/crafting/writing area to keep the creative energy flowing.

Sea salt

A small jar or bottle with top

Orange peel

Carnelian chips

Citrine chips

Chrysanthemum or chamomile flowers

Calendula herb

Fire and Focus Oil (see page 124)

Spill your salt on your table or workspace, and make a small hole in the middle with your fingers. Place your jar or bottle in the center of the salt circle. This will act like a barrier to concentrate the energy as much as we can.

Repeat the same affirmation for each ingredient as you add each to the jar or bottle. By the end of the spell, you should have said it at least seven times total. Say: *"Solar power, give me energy. Your light and power radiate through me, into this jar. So, mote it be."*

Add your orange peel, then your carnelian chips. Next the citrine, then chrysanthemum with your calendula flowers. Last is going to be a few drops of your Fire and Focus Oil.

Once everything is all up in there, pop the top of the jar back on and say the affirmation again twice.

When not in use, keep your jar near your bathroom or on your altar. When you feel the need for an extra charged surge of energy, hold the jar in your hands for sixty-six seconds. (Yes, you can count to sixty-six in your head; it'll help you stay focused on what you're doing, as well.) Recharge every two to four weeks in the sunlight.

MENTAL "WINDOWS UPDATE" TEA

JUST LIKE YOUR spaces need to be reset every once in a while, so does your brain. That's where this tea comes in.

1 tablespoon (15 g) lemongrass

1 teaspoon (5 g) rosemary

1 tablespoon (15 g) calendula

1 teaspoon (5 g) grated orange peel

Empty tea bag or sachet

Pen and paper

Tea cup (clear is recommended)

Begin by charging the herbs and adding them into the tea bag. Hold each herb in your hand before adding them to the sachet and say the following affirmation: *"Reset my mental energy. Reset my social battery. Reset my will to continue my journey."*

Once your bag is full, use the pen and paper to make a sigil out of the word "reset" (see page 29 for more on sigils). Place your sigil underneath your cup while its brewing.

Brew your tea. You can brew it with hot water for two to three minutes or place it in your fridge for three to four hours for a cold brew. Add in honey or sugar while stirring counterclockwise to get rid of any trash vibes. Then stir clockwise twice to bring back the good energy.

Drink your tea like you normally would. When you're finished, discard everything in a trash receptacle located outside of your home.

ZERO-SPOON *spell*

Make an energy playlist to use as a sound spell when you're just not feeling life.

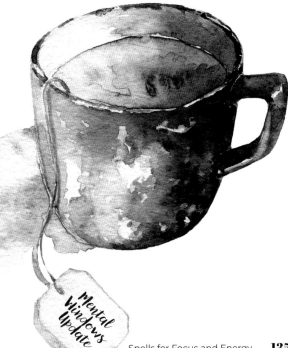

CREATIVE INSPIRATION RITUAL

CREATIVITY DOESN'T NECESSARILY mean art, drawing, or writing. You can be creative in any job you have. Need to come up with ways to start a new project? Creativity. Have to find a new way to accomplish a task and make it more efficient? That's also creativity. You use creativity all of the time in your personal and work life, so why not get a helping hand from this inspirational ritual?

Don't get overwhelmed with this one. It's as straightforward as all my other spells even though it seems long. Just take it one step at a time.

Fire and Focus Oil (see page 124)
1 white candle
1 orange candle
1 yellow candle
Frankincense incense
Citrine chunk
Red jasper chunk
Carnelian chunk (raw chunk preferred but not required)
Sea salt
Feather
Notebook and pen

This spell takes place outside. Start by dressing your candles. Rub a small amount of Fire and Focus Oil onto each candle. Do this step before going outside.

Once outside, light your incense and place it in front of you. Set your candles around the incense in a triangle formation. Place your crystals in between the candles to make a full circle around the incense. Use your sea salt to fill in the gaps between your items.

Use your feather to fan the smoke of the incense toward you. If you have asthma or the smoke bothers you, you can fan it onto your notebook instead.

Do this for about two to three minutes while focusing on the fire coming from the candles. If you're not able to focus the entire time, it's totally fine. Our minds wander naturally, but pay attention to where your thoughts take you.

Once ideas start popping up in your head, write them down. Write anything you think of down. Even if it's an incomplete thought or it literally just doesn't make sense. WRITE IT ALL DOWN. Keep writing until your smoke goes out or your candles are done.

Once your candles have cooled, throw them in the trash. The next day, revisit your notebook and try to complete the thoughts you had. It should come pretty easily since your subconscious had all night to think about it without you even noticing.

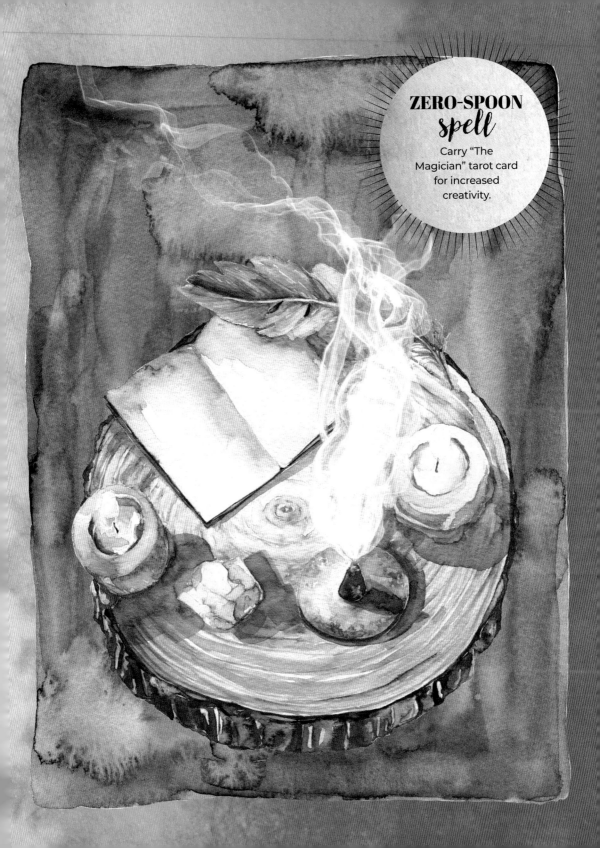

ZERO-SPOON *spell*

Carry "The Magician" tarot card for increased creativity.

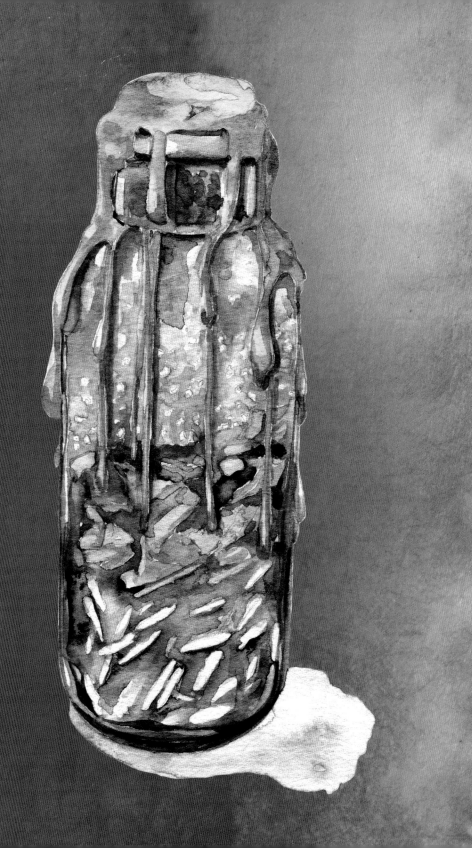

6

SPELLS FOR
money +
abundance

In many magical and spiritual groups, the word
"abundance" is used, literally, all the fucking time. There
are a shit ton of spells and rituals out there aimed at
creating abundance.

Abundance just means to have a lot of something. We often associate it with having a lot of money or easy access to it, but the term can also refer to being able to easily meet one's basic necessities, having an abundance of joy and happiness, or having plenty of opportunities. You can use abundance magic to open doors, draw clients to your business, make more money, or lure a wealth of love, happiness, and friendship into your life. If we wanted to get super basic with it, abundance just means the absence of lack. You lack nothing, because you already have what you need to make your dreams a reality.

Money is pure energy. When we're financially stressed or pressed, it drastically affects our energy, which is why I included a few money spells in this book to help boost your efforts. But mindset is important here, too. Your actions are not as important as the energy you put into them. Spend in love instead of fear. When you spend out of fear that the money won't come back, you block your blessings. This doesn't mean go wild and spend all the money in your account. It just means don't let your concern about indulging in your favorite things prevent you from enjoying your financial blessings.

Remember that witchcraft only works when you do. You can't expect money to fall from the sky if you're chilling on the couch watching TV. In this economy, we need all the help we can get, magical AND mundane, especially when we're questioning our existence in this dystopian consumer capitalist world. (If everything goes according to plan, we'll take over the 1 percent with this chapter. Okay, probably not but let's just keep that energy as we continue.)

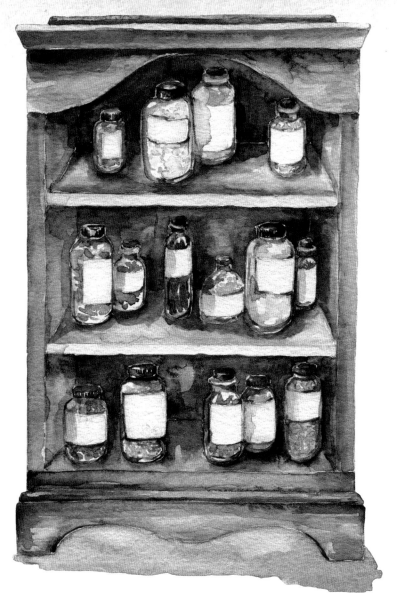

MATERIALS AND CORRESPONDENCES FOR LAZY WITCH
abundance magic

Here are the correspondences we'll use in this chapter.
As you can see, we're focusing on money, abundance, wealth,
and luck as our main intentions.

CORRESPONDENCES FOR MONEY, ABUNDANCE, WEALTH, AND LUCK

	Money	Abundance	Wealth	Luck
Moon Phase	Full, waxing	Full, waxing	Full, waxing	Waxing
Zodiac	Gemini	Virgo	Taurus	No substitute
Tarot Card	Pentacles	Pentacles	The Wheel of Fortune	The Wheel of Fortune
Colors	Copper, gold, green, silver	Gold, green, orange	Gold, green, purple	Blue, green, orange, purple
Herbs, Plants, and Flowers	Cedar, olive leaf, patchouli, chamomile, comfrey, dandelion, lemon balm, peppermint, vervain, cinnamon, galangal, pine	Myrrh, elder, oak, olive, pine, basil, bergamot, chamomile, St. John's wort, vervain, allspice, cinnamon, clove, galangal, ginger, nutmeg, patchouli	Apple, cedar, olive, pine, pomegranate, basil, chamomile, clove, comfrey, jasmine, cinnamon, galangal, myrrh, patchouli	Cedar, oak, pomegranate, chamomile, clove, jasmine, peppermint, rose, yarrow, anise, galangal, ginger, patchouli, nettle, sandalwood, star anise

And here's your list of materials,

along with their substitutions.

PLANTS, HERBS, AND FLOWERS

Ingredient	Substitution
Basil	Thyme
Bay leaf	Spell paper
Chamomile	Lemongrass
Cinnamon	Clove
Frankincense	Myrrh
Ginger	Comfrey
Juniper berry	Elderberry
Lemongrass	Lemon balm
Orange peel	Lemon peel
Orris root	Galangal root
Patchouli	Vervain
Peppermint	Spearmint
Pine needle	Olive leaf
Rice	No substitute
Sea salt	Table salt

CARRIER OILS AND ESSENTIAL OILS

Ingredient	Substitution
Basil essential oil	Basil
Olive oil	Sunflower oil
Patchouli essential oil	Patchouli

CRYSTALS AND GEMSTONES

Ingredient	Substitution
Green aventurine (chips or tumbles)	Green calcite
Moss agate (chips or tumbles)	Tree agate
Pyrite (chips or tumbles)	Citrine

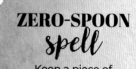

ZERO-SPOON spell

Keep a piece of green aventurine in your pocket for luck.

BASIC TEALIGHTS, SIGILS, AND OIL BLENDS
abundance spellwork

Here are your basic tealights, sigils, and oils for abundance spellwork. The Abundance and Money Oil (page 144) will be used on repeat, so I recommend making that one in advance.

TWO-INGREDIENT TEALIGHTS FOR MONEY AND ABUNDANCE

REMEMBER TO SET your intentions.

Tealight

Herbs and Crystals:

- Money: peppermint and citrine chips
- Success: orange peel and carnelian chips
- Abundance: rosemary and peppermint chips

Light the tealight, and let the wax melt a bit. Blow it out when you have a melty surface.

Sprinkle your herbs and chips on top of the melted wax, being careful and cautious NOT to let the herbs near the flame. Use immediately or save for later.

ABUNDANCE SIGILS AND WHERE TO DRAW THEM

CREATE A SIGIL based on your intentions for abundance and use them as follows (for full instructions on how to make a sigil, see Chapter 1, page 29):

- Write "MONEY" on the inside of your wallet or purse.
- Draw "SUCCESS" on the bottom of your keyboard (you can also make the sigil on sticker paper and stick that directly on your laptop).
- Add "WEALTH" underneath your front door mat.

ABUNDANCE AND MONEY OIL

THIS ABUNDANCE AND MONEY OIL will help you with money, success, goals, dreams, finance, business adventures, career changes, and so on. Use on candles, to anoint yourself, in baths, sprays, spell jars, and so much more.

4 ounces (120 ml) olive oil

Lemongrass

Peppermint

Basil

Green aventurine chips

30 drops of basil essential oil

4-ounce (120-ml) dropper bottle

For this specific oil, we'll infuse the herbs listed above using heat. Now, usually, I fucking hate using the stove to make oils. I'd much rather let it sit for a few weeks in a cool, dark place; however, to make her as potent as we can, we will use the stove.

Pour the olive oil into the pot, and set the pot on the stove over low heat.

Sprinkle the herbs into the pot one by one, telling each one why they're there as you do:

"Lemongrass, bring me prosperity.
Peppermint, bring me abundance.
Basil, bring me wealth."

Let your herbs sit in your oil for about 5 to 10 minutes. You don't want them to start simmering; you just need them to heat up.

Turn your stove off, and leave the herbs to infuse for about an hour.

Once the oil is completely cooled, you can decide whether you'd like to strain the herbs out or if you want to leave them in there. That choice is totally up to you. If you leave the herbs in, you'll essentially infuse the oil for its entire shelf life; my preferences is to leave them. The only pro to straining is prolonging the shelf life. With the herbs, it is about a month or two. Without, you can keep it on your altar for up to six months.

When the oil is infused, add the green aventurine to the dropper oil. Say: *"Green like money, green like go, green surrounds me from head to toe."*

Add the basil essential oil and then pour the infused oil mixture into the bottle. Remember to shake before each use to wake that magic up a bit.

LAZY WITCH SPELLS AND RITUALS FOR
money + abundance

PROSPERITY INCENSE BLEND

INCENSE CONES AND sticks are pretty technical and hard to make, which is why I absolutely adore loose incense. This prosperity incense can be customized to match your current intent by simply waving your hand over it and saying a short affirmation.

Frankincense

Peppermint

Ginger

The smallest pinch ever of cinnamon

Mortar and pestle (see note)

Container

Cauldron

Charcoal tab

Combine your frankincense, peppermint, ginger, and cinnamon in your mortar and pestle. Grind it up until you have a powder consistency.

Once that bitch is dusty, wave your hand over it and recite the following, three times: *"Universe, grant me the power to attract prosperity. Smoke and dust turn to prosperity as they must. So it is said, so it shall be."*

Transfer to a container and store for up to six months.

To use, light a piece of charcoal, and sprinkle a pinch of your incense right on top.

Note: If you don't have the time, patience, and energy to grind shit up, you can use a coffee bean grinder, but make sure you NEVER use it for food afterwards. Frankincense is NOT good for ingestion.

THE MOST BASIC PROSPERITY SPELL

"I will always have enough money."
"I am filled with the energy of abundance."
"I am open to limitless possibility."

Carving tool

1 green candle

Paintbrush

Abundance and Money Oil (see page 144)

Gold candle holder (optional)

Before you begin the spell, choose one word that represents your intention and use your carving tool to carve it into your candle and carving tool. You can use Money, Luck, Abundance, Prosperity, Wealth, or choose one of your own. If you don't want to write the actual word, feel free to use a sigil instead (see page 29).

Use a paintbrush to brush a small amount of the Money and Abundance Oil onto the candle. (You can use your bare hands, but you might be smelling the oil on them for the next three days because that shit is potent as fuck.)

Find a place where no one will interrupt you and settle down. Place your candle directly in front of you and light her up. Breathe in through your mouth for eight counts, hold for four, breathe out through your mouth for eight. Do this three times total—or, you know, just meditate if you have the mental capacity to do so. More power to ya, because I simply cannot sit still for long enough.

Start chanting your chosen affirmation. As you chant, start to visualize your life after this spell. Visualize yourself with all of the wealth you can imagine. Visualize your house, your car, your partner, your health. What will that look like? What color is your hair? How does the air smell? What does the ground feel like? Visualize yourself as if the abundance you're seeking has already manifested itself.

Repeat the chant and visualization until the candle is completely gone.

Discard the leftovers in the trash (inside your house or outside—this time it doesn't matter).

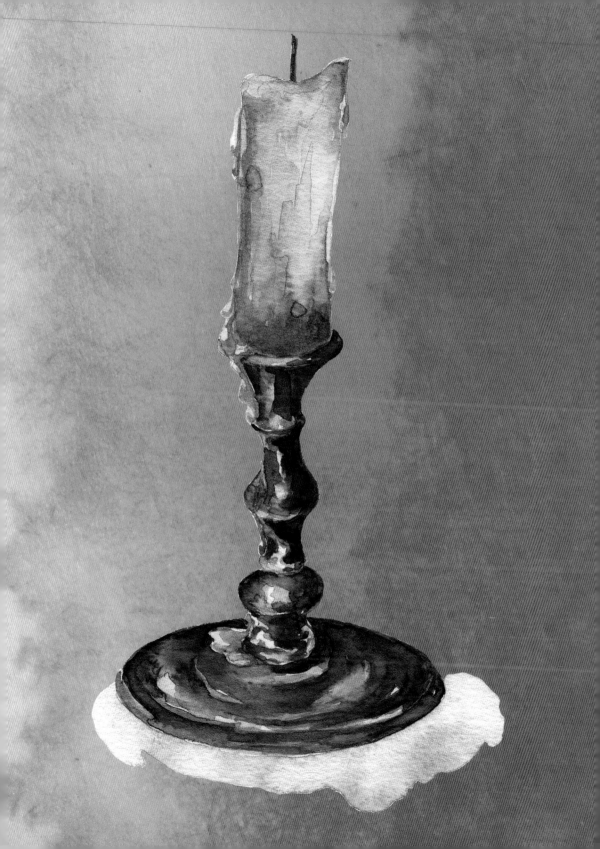

HEALTH AND WEALTH SPELL JAR

SPELL JARS ARE easy and effective as fuck. I've done this spell every single time I needed some extra cash for a side project, and it never disappoints.

1 green candle

Paper and pen

Pyrite sand

A jar with a cork

Rice

Peppermint

Orris root

Lemongrass

Basil

A small key to "open opportunity" (optional)

Light your candle.

Grab paper and a pen and write exactly what you want. Whatever that may be, remember to be as specific as you can. You want money and health to come in, not to be served an eviction notice while you're in the hospital.

Burn a small corner of your paper on your candle to activate it.

Put your paper to the side and start filling your jar. Add the pyrite sand first, then the rice and leave the herbs for last. Every time you add something to your jar, recite the following affirmation: *"I am happy, healthy, wealthy, and wise. Everything is always working out for me. My life is unfolding in divine order."*

Last, add your paper. Rip it up into pieces that are small enough to fit in the jar. Always rip toward you for this one. You want that energy coming in, not going out.

Close your jar and seal with wax from the lighted candle.

Keep your jar on your altar or in your purse/backpack.

Recharge in the sunlight every week.

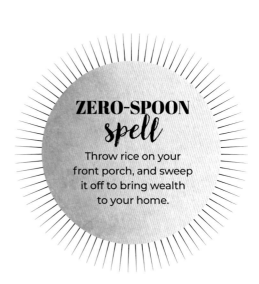

ZERO-SPOON
spell

Throw rice on your front porch, and sweep it off to bring wealth to your home.

BILLS AND SHIT

THIS SPELL IS meant to help your bills disappear—in a metaphorical sense, of course. The goal with this spell is to manifest money in your life faster so your bills are covered. Note that the candle in this spell needs to be lit for fifteen minutes, once a day, for seven days. You don't need a whole pillar, but you do need it to last that long, so a large taper or even an oversized tealight should work as well.

A copy of the bill in question

Lighter

Charcoal tablets

Cauldron

Pine needles

Cinnamon (see note)

1 green pillar candle

Abundance and Money Oil (see page 144)

First, an important warning: Do not use your original bill for this spell. Use a copy. Unless you can get it online, in which case, go wild. Now, let's burn some shit.

Light the charcoal and put it in your cauldron. Add a pinch of pine needles to the cauldron. It should start smoking right away.

Rip the copy of your bill into pieces small enough to fit into your cauldron safely. Add each piece of the bill while repeating: *"This bill is paid. This bill is paid. This bill is paid."*

Once you have all your papers in, add a pinch of cinnamon. (Cinnamon can be an irritant if burned too often; if it bothers you, use dried mint leaves.) Let the charcoal go out all the way, and make sure your cauldron has cooled down before trying to touch it. If you're impatient like I am, use oven gloves at your own risk.

Dress your candle with a small amount of the Abundance and Money Oil. You can carve a money sigil on the candle or you can "draw" it with the oil, if you want. Sprinkle the ashes from your cauldron onto the candle; the oil should help it stick really well.

Light your candle. Visualize the bill, why you need to pay it, and why it's important. Wave your hand over the candle (don't fucking burn yourself, though) while saying: *"The candle burns and lights the way. Money coming, money paid."*

Let the candle burn for about fifteen minutes, then blow it out. Repeat this spell every day for seven days. On the seventh day, you can either discard the candle or continue to burn it at the same time of the month if the bill is repetitive.

THE MONEY BOWL

I FUCKING LOVE MONEY BOWLS, Y'ALL. No seriously, I've made so many. Money bowls are so easy to throw together and very easy to upkeep, so they're the perfect spell for a crazy, shitty day when you need a little extra help in the financial department.

Before you begin, know that you don't need all the herbs I listed in the spell. An ideal money bowl includes anywhere from four to ten herbs. These are my personal money bowl ingredients, tried and true, but the amounts you use in your spell are up to you.

Peppermint

Orris root

Pine needle

Ginger

Orange peel

Lemongrass

Chamomile buds

Patchouli

Green aventurine (chips or tumbles)

Pyrite (chips or tumbles)

Moss agate (chips or tumbles)

Gold flakes

Fake dollar bills (see note)

A pretty bowl (I usually stick with wood)

Take a moment to get into the right headspace. You can do this by lighting a candle or incense, doing a breathing or meditation exercise, or just sit there until your intuition says it's time. Once you're ready, you can begin.

First add the herbs to the bowl, then the crystals, then your extras. Remember, don't freak the fuck out if you don't have EVERYTHING I listed. You could literally use three herbs and one crystal without messing up the bowl. Your intention is the main ingredient.

As you add each item to the bowl, tell it why the fuck it's there. You can use your own associations or, if repetitive thinking is easier for you, you can use the following chant and repeat it throughout the whole process: *"Money and wealth, luck and prosperity. Herbs and crystals bring me plenty. Success is drawn to me by the many. So it is said, so it shall be. Harm to none, good for me."*

The last thing to go in your bowl should be the fake money.

Once you're happy with your bowl, it's time to give it its first meal. Place the bowl somewhere near the front door. If you live with roommates, keep the bowl on your desk. Take any coin you have and toss it in. Repeat the chant from earlier.

To keep it alive, feed it every day with real coins (in your desired currency, of course). This is why placing it by the front door is perfect; you can't forget if you see it every time.

You can keep feeding the same bowl for months without needing to refresh it. However, if you feel the energy is off or the money isn't moneying correctly, you can recharge your bowl in the sunlight.

Extra credit: You can add resin to your bowl to make it a permanent piece of décor in your home. Yes, bitch! Just pour a small amount of the resin (follow the directions provided) into the bowl before you begin. Swirl it around the bottom to make a coating. After you've added your ingredients, wait about three to four hours and then come back with more resin. Pour it all over everything until it's completely submerged. Let it cure for for a couple of days and then use it like normal. Resin will yellow in the sunlight, so to recharge you'll need to use the moonlight.

Note: Sorry, ripping up real money is illegal unless you have special permission from our government. If you don't want to use fake money, grab a bay leaf and draw a money sigil on that bitch.

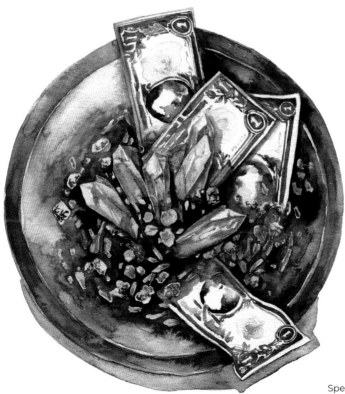

ABUNDANCE FOOT SOAK

WASHING YOUR HANDS with chamomile tea is an old superstition that we're basically taking to the next level. Why did I switch it to feet instead of hands? Science. Mostly everyone has seen the "potato in your socks" trick to help detox your entire body, right? So, if we take that and use the theory that we can also add in energy to our entire body through our feet, we get a money foot soak.

6 bay leaves

Pen or marker

4 parts sea salt

Bowl

1 part chamomile

1 part lemongrass

1 part pine

1 ounce (28 ml) olive oil

30 drops of patchouli essential oil

16-ounce (475-ml) jar or container

Food-safe gold flakes (optional)

Start with your bay leaves. Write an intention on each leaf. For this spell, you could use Money, Abundance, Luck, Prosperity, Good Health, or Success. You can write the whole word, make up an abbreviation, or make a sigil (see page 29).

Add the sea salt to your bowl. Say: *"Salt, cleanse my energy from anything no longer serving me."*

Next, add the herbs and say: *"Herbs and plants, enhance my prosperity in all aspects of my life."*

Hold your bay leaves directly above the bowl, and crush them before throwing them in. Pour in the olive oil and add your essential oil. Mix super, super well, going clockwise.

Transfer the mix to your jar container. (Pro tip: Stick a piece of citrine in the jar with your soak to have it be super charged every time.)

To use, grab a bucket or fill your tub with warm water (or hot— I don't know what you're into).

You don't need to use a specific amount of this soak for it to work. I know not everyone has access to unlimited materials, but if you can, I like to use a full cup when I do this ritual. Maybe a cup and a half if I'm feeling crazy.

Add the blend to the water. Soak your feet until the water starts to get lukewarm/cold.

While your feet are soaking, visualize what these salts are meant to bring into your life.

If you want money, what's your bank account going to look like?
If you want health, what activities would you be able to do?
If you want friendships and relationships, what are they like?

When you're done, toss the water outside of your house because it essentially soaked up all the unlucky, gross energy from the bottoms of your feet. You don't want that inside y'all.

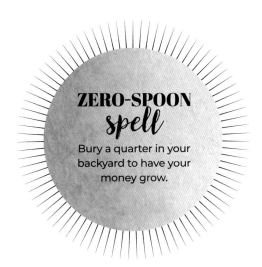

ZERO-SPOON
spell
Bury a quarter in your backyard to have your money grow.

ZERO-SPOON
spell

Draw a "luck" sigil on your résumé with your finger to help you get that job, you boss-ass bitch.

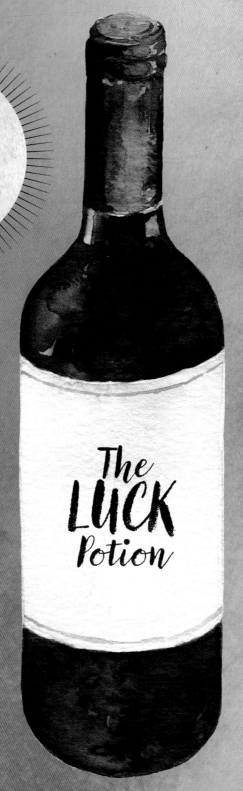

The
LUCK
Potion

THE LUCK POTION

NOT ONLY DOES this spell make a fire ass sangria, but it also combines the intentions of these fruits and spices to make a potion that brings good luck, wealth, and success. For this spell, we'll use alcohol. If you are not of legal drinking age, have a condition that does not allow you to drink, or you simply just hate liquor, you can use grape juice. There are no other substitutions for this recipe. I can't promise it'll taste good if you substitute any of the ingredients so do it at your own risk, babe.

Empty pitcher or bottle

6 ounces (175 ml) pomegranate juice

6 ounces (175 ml) orange juice

2 oranges, sliced

10 strawberries, halved

10 blackberries

3 cinnamon sticks

1 bottle of red wine (see note)

It's easiest to make everything directly in the pitcher so you don't have hella dishes to wash. (Seems like a lot.)

Add all ingredients to the pitcher except the red wine. Wave your hand over the pitcher and say: *"Bring me luck, bring me wealth. Bring me money and good health. Bring me everything I deserve, everything that is on this earth. So mote it be."*

Add your red wine in last and stir.

Stick your potion in the fridge overnight (for at least eight hours), and drink whenever you want. The shelf life for this potion is three days so be sure to make it right before drinking. You can strain out the fruits and spices to extend the shelf life to 4 days. Pro tip: Share this potion with your friends (with magical consent, of course) and make it a whole event.

Note: If you're using alcohol for this spell, try a pinot noir since it's such a light red wine. If you're not using alcohol, substitute it for grape juice. Same properties, no hangover.

EARTH SPELL FOR ABUNDANCE

THIS SPELL IS a three-spoon spell mostly because you're going to have to go outside. I know, it's a lot. You've got this, though. The earth embodies all intentions having to do with agriculture, business, growth, money, prosperity, strength, success, and wealth. In this spell, you'll literally use the earth as an oven to grow your prosperity and success.

Paper and pencil
(see note)

Peppermint

Orris root

Ginger

Green aventurine
chips

Grab your paper and pencil because it's time to write. Write everything you want to come to you. Keep it simple, make it detailed—the choice is yours. The earth will amplify your intention for you.

Now, use the paper as your vessel. Sprinkle the herbs in the middle of your paper. You can either fold it to keep the herbs inside or crumble it up. Either way, you want the herbs inside of the paper.

Go in your backyard (or front yard, or to a random forest) and dig a hole. It doesn't need to be 8 feet deep or 10 feet wide. Just a lil' hole, deep enough to cover the paper. Place your herb paper pouch in the hole, and toss your green aventurine on top.

Cover the hole with dirt and leave it alone.

Go on about your life, and let the earth send your message out into the universe.

Extra credit: Throw some basil or wildflower seeds (or whatever is native to your land) in the paper along with your herbs. It's an easy way to show gratitude to the earth for helping you out with this spell.

Note: Almost all paper is biodegradable with the exception of those that are coated or laminated. Use handmade paper to be extra earth-friendly. Pens and markers also sometime make paper harder to break down, which is why I said "pencil" specifically in this spell.

about the author

Born and raised in Tampa, Florida (with a detour in Atlanta, Georgia), **Andrea Samayoa** has been a practicing witch for seven years. She started Moon Street Kits, an Etsy shop and accompanying TikTok channel, in 2020 with the goal of making her space accessible to beginners and to end the stigma behind witchcraft. Her page has been a haven for beginners and generational witches alike who love her "no bullshit" approach that makes it easy for viewers to follow her tutorials and still feel like they're connecting with a real person with realistic goals.

index